Bedtime

MW01233304

for

Stressed Out Adults

Learn the Power of Visualization, Relieve Worries, Reduce Anxiety, Heal Insomnia, and Fall Asleep Deeply with a Smile.

By

Diana Shelby

Table of Contents

Introduction

Hey, hi, nice to meet you.

Thank you for choosing my book.

I hope you will allow me to take you by the hand to make a nice regenerating journey together, and always keep in mind that my goal is only one: to make you feel good.

For some of us it is strange that now that we are adults, we need to listen bedtime stories, and yet, trust me, we all need it more than we think, only many of us don't know it, or don't want to admit it.

Do you remember when, as children, mom, dad, or a babysitter used to tell us fairy tales before we went to sleep to put us into a deep sleep?
Wasn't that one of the most relaxing moments of our childhood?

Oh, at that time I waited for the bedtime story with such trepidation, I loved so much to immerse myself in other worlds

5

while crouching comfortably in my bed, I was as if relieved from all negative thoughts - even children have their own stress, didn't you know that? - and I was finally able to relax.

Before we start with our stories though, please allow me to briefly tell you my experience.

I was going through a particularly stressed period, everything was going badly, it seemed that the world was angry with me and that my life was taking a wrong turn.

One evening, coming home from a day at work where problems were hitting me like I was the center of the target of a game of darts, I felt the extreme need for something to comfort me, to be transported to a shelter away from everything, in a world where nothing and nobody could hurt my person.

How to do it? I was asking me.

I didn't want to sit for hours in front of the TV inebriating myself with talk shows or TV series that manipulate your brain to the point of making you almost addicted, I absolutely didn't want to binge on junk food, and it wouldn't make sense to pour me something alcoholic that would only make me feel worse later on, and I didn't want to bore my family or some friends with my problems. If it's true that sometimes a friendly word is what can lift our mood, when fatigue overwhelms everything it's hard to even focus on a dialogue, pick up a phone and explain to someone on the other end of the line why our boss is such an asshole, or why you think your partner is cheating on you, or why it's hard to raise children and do the math at the end of the month. Or maybe, why not, you can be furious just for a wrong haircut, for finding the car door scratched, or for making a plant die. Regardless of the cause or the height of our fall, we have accused the blow, and when you have a bruise, we would like nothing more than a magic balm that soothes the pain and makes the marks disappear quickly.

Tell me, am I wrong?

No, I do not think so.

Well, that evening I was exactly looking for a soothing balm for my bruises. I came by to say good night to my children, to tuck them in and make sure they were comfortable and ready for sleep. Before turning off the bedroom light, my eye fell on the book that my little girl, already deeply asleep, had left open on the bedside table next to her. On one page there was an illustration of a huge orange pumpkin, painted in watercolor, rolling unstoppably from the countryside to a village, chased by farmers. What a nice image! I immediately thought. So, I grabbed my daughter's book and took it to my room. I slipped into bed and started flipping through the pages of those bedtime stories, full of positive and reassuring characters and settings, of heroes, of enchanted castles, of heavenly places where people lived happily and carefree.

Oh, what a jump into the past!

That night I felt good, I fell asleep with a serenity that I had forgotten, without difficulty in turning off the continuous flow of thoughts, without focusing on missed opportunities in my life or those I might miss in the future, melting away the stress accumulated at work and in the family thanks to relaxing words, fantastic worlds, positivity and beautiful things. I was so relieved by the anxiety that normally crushed me against the pillow, that I did not even realize that I had dozed off halfway through the story, completely relieved.

Now I would like to be able to spread this benefit to you too, make you return to the innocence of childhood, or think like a child, to find that deep sleep that is the best cure for everything.

I only ask you to take the right approach and let yourself go to what you will be offered, otherwise, as they say in fairy tales, the spell will not work!

Enjoy your reading.

Chapter 1 Autumn Walk

Here we are, ready for the first story.

Put yourself in a comfortable position, or even better it would be in your favorite position, inside your cozy bed or maybe on the sofa with a wrap-around blanket and a soft pillow under your head.

Relax, let yourself go, just focus on the story, and forget everything else. Leave the bad things out, they are not part of you now.

If it is already night, it is important that you have already completed your good night routine. I know it is usually done by children, but it is essential that adults also have their own reassuring routine, such as washing their face with a specific detergent, brushing their teeth, peeing and drinking a sip of water. These are simple but habitual steps, and habits are sometimes among those sensations that make us feel safe and sheltered.

Now imagine that it is the end of October, a month that has arrived quickly, bringing with it a taste of winter and that unique autumn atmosphere.

Autumn advances slowly but inexorably creeps in, without excesses. It has a taste of old things, partly neglected, more often forgotten.

Autumn resembles a rare lace, aged by time and perhaps a little yellowed, hidden in a dusty trunk of a few centuries ago. Yet, it is enough to recover it and observe it without haste to understand its eternal, immutable beauty, and to grasp, amazed and moved, its precious, unreachable enchantment.

Autumn smells of light and thin rain, of faded memories, of mud and fog that takes refuge outside the big cities.

Autumn is a scent of good things, of the first hot chocolates, of a good, sweet liqueur, of good mushrooms that smell of fresh earth, of sweet and juicy grapes, of pomegranate a bit bitter and a bit sweet and finally of the inevitable floury chestnuts.

The real enchantment of this season, however, is in its colors, unique colors that fill our eyes with wonder wherever we look.

So, imagine having as much time as you want for an autumn walk

You are wearing a warm coat and do not feel any cold.

It's a day without commitments, the atmosphere is perfect, and no one will come to disturb you, you don't have any agenda with you, no phone or pager, it's a moment all yours, only yours.

You walk along an alley with white gravel, it is very pleasant the noise that your footsteps make on small pebbles.

Suddenly, you put your hand in your pocket and you discover that you have a key with you, it's a special key, quite big, with a gothic coat of arms on top.

You keep walking a little longer and the gravel starts to leave room under your feet for a carpet of yellow leaves. You go on, relaxing and enjoying the fresh and crisp air, until you come across an extremely high and rusty gate.

In front of your eyes there is a big lock, hey, don't you have a key?

Of course, I do.

Take your gothic key out of your pocket and try to insert it into the patch. Although the gate is rusty and old made, extremely high and with spikes on the top, the key turns easily by triggering the opening of the lock.

The gate is of those fascinating, rare, and ancient, and with a particular creaking invites you to enter a beautiful park, an unknown and pleasant place, where only you can enter.

The air is pungent, but you like it to mess up your hair.

The trees all around lose their leaves and become bare and unadorned. Everywhere they have taken on amazing colors, nature has such an infinite palette of colors in shades of brown, golden and orange yellows, brick or rust, or red and scarlet purple of some creepers that any painter would make fake cards to be able to recreate those colors. Even the pines that are evergreens have brown bangs. On the bark the resin is amber and viscous. The leaves, falling from the highest branches, spin and fall to the ground forming a soft carpet.

Continue your quiet walk through the park, the driest leaves crackle like wood in the fireplace. There is no other noise.

The morning dew impresses the grass of the lawn spared by the foliage.

Imagine now being attracted by a yellow leaf. A tender, star-shaped leaf, attached to its twig only by a fragile little leg. This leaf trembles all morning to evening, and at night she can't even close her eyes because of the cold shivers.

The parent tree watches and comforts her with infinite patience, without ever getting tired, repeating to her: "You don't want to let yourself fall, you are afraid, you don't want to get confused with the other leaves and rot in the ground, but you don't understand that the falling leaves are not lost. Little leaves like you and of all shapes and colors fall into the ground to help a new seedling or flower to grow, to keep the roots of an old tree warm or to provide bedding for the animals in the stables. Pretty as you are in addition, my little leaf, you could also be collected by a child and become one of its precious treasures. Perhaps a maiden with a romantic soul could lay you down to rest between the pages of a book and keep you as a special memory.

Hearing these words, the little leaf every time has a motion of emotion and in the end, she is convinced that there is a need for her, so at the first gust of wind, she lets herself be carried away.

The first snow that falls will cover her and help her to become part of the ground: there she will know a new life and will not feel lonely anymore.

Isn't it true that sometimes falls can be good for us?

Continuing further on the walk, you arrive at the foot of a huge chestnut tree, it is a majestic and imposing tree, almost five centuries old. It has an exceptionally large and solid trunk, it communicates stability and solidity, and its huge branches seem to communicate an embrace.

By instinct, the hug to the trunk of the great chestnut tree is replaced with momentum.

Many of us, at some point in our lives, have experienced the wonderful feeling of hugging a tree. It is a primordial instinct that we feel extraordinarily strong especially as children, even if with advancing age the need to let ourselves go to this spontaneous union with nature is diminishing more and more. In this park nobody sees you and you are free to do even those things that would make you feel embarrassed elsewhere, so if you want to hug a tree you can do it.

It is like embracing an old man, the wrinkled rind, hard to the touch, so many things to tell. Drops of resin glisten on its surface, pieces of bark flake under your fingers.

According to many studies, trees are a source of emotional and physical healing, they absorb and preserve all the energy of the cosmos, and by embracing them we absorb all their benefit.

There are many ancient legends about how the chestnut tree "got" its fruits. In a distant time, the chestnut tree was always incredibly sad because, unlike other trees, it had no fruits to give to children. For this reason, one day he went to the Green Fairy expressing the desire to have fruits too, but the Fairy asked him to wait a year. And so, just in those days of waiting, the chestnut tree found himself helping a family of hedgehogs that ran away from a pack of dogs, making them climb on its branches to hide them from view. After this altruistic and heartfelt gesture, the Green Fairy decided to reward the tree and to remember what happened she gave him chestnuts enclosed in green hedgehogs.

Another legend, however, explains why the chestnuts are wrapped in hedgehogs. It seems that, in order to escape the freezing cold of winter, the chestnut tree's fruits asked for protection, a kind of natural blanket not to continue to suffer the low temperatures. And here, too, appear the little animals from the spines. According to legend, in fact, the hedgehogs, pitiless by the suffering of the chestnuts, climbed along the branches of the tree and wrapped them, leaving their fur made of chestnut spines, a warm and protective blanket against the cold.

Is it not true that we all often protect ourselves with a blanket of spines?

Do you know that old legend about the three sisters' chestnuts?

Oh, it's a very beautiful story.

In a thorny hedgehog were locked three chestnuts: three twin sisters.

Grow up and grow up, push, and push, one fine day the hedgehog opened up. The chestnuts, one after the other, fell. The two sisters who grew to the right and left of the hedgehog were beautiful, with a curved, shiny back and a feather on top. Instead, the little sister who grew up in the middle had remained a little chestnut. The woman who did the gathering did not want it. She took the two beautiful little sisters and left her in the woods alone and sad.

The two beautiful sisters went out into the world. One was cooked in the frying pan and became golden and fragrant. A greedy child took her; he opened his mouth wide and... uh! The first chestnut was no more.

The second one ended up in a confectioner's basket. The confectioner peeled it, cooked it in sugar, put it to dry. It had become overly sweet and sparkling. A little girl who had a little mouth that looked like a rose bought it: she cut it into tiny little pieces. Then the little pieces disappeared, one by one, in that little rose mouth: and the second chestnut was no more.

The third chestnut, poor thing, so alone in the woods, complained to the crickets and the other animals: uh, my little sisters have been around the world and I'm staying here alone, in the thick forest, in the cold of winter, and under the snow to rot.
But, as if by magic, she didn't rot.

Little by little she felt something alive germinating inside her little body. A little white, strong root began to push itself downwards, into the earth. A tender little green plant began to sprout upwards, looking for sunlight.

Now, the smallest, the most modest of the three twin sisters has become a beautiful chestnut tree, full of hedgehogs, squirrels, and nests.

You hear something moving shortly afterwards near your feet, and you discover that it is just a hedgehog walking like you in the park. A small and extremely cute little animal, but above all strong and definitely unique.

Just behind him, you see a little squirrel with reddish colors running amazingly fast to bring an acorn into the den.

It seems that these little animals know exactly what to do and where to go, better than many human beings.

Following the squirrel your eyes cross a magnificent and majestic Gingko biloba tree, it is of breathtaking beauty. Normally its small leaves with the characteristic appearance of a fan, or whale tail, or almost heart-shaped, are a beautiful bright green, but in winter they are tinged with a fabulous golden yellow. This is a very ancient tree, a sort of "living fossil" whose species is certainly the oldest on earth.

In oriental tradition the Ginkgo is a metaphor of coincidence between opposites and symbolizes the immutability of things. It is said to have magical powers and to be able to ward off evil spirits: that is why it was planted near temples and places of worship.

Imagine that you can place the palm of your hand on the trunk of this magnificent ancient gift that nature has handed down to us, it will help you ward off all malice and negativity and fill your heart with beauty.

Feel the connection with it and the surrounding nature. The Ginkgo watches over you.

Now, thanks also to the beneficial influence of Ginkgo, we can let ourselves go for a break. Sometimes all we need is a little break, and we feel better right away.

Near the majestic old tree there is a comfortable bench. It looks like one of those movie benches, inviting and accommodating, clean, with some decorations on the top and sides. I have always seen them as sofas in those living rooms that are gardens or parks. Here no one will come to disturb your peace or claim a little space next to you, you can get comfortable, legs open or crossed, or even lie down if you feel like it. No one will look at you crooked, and the bench is clean.

Imagine you are sitting down and looking up at the sky.

You will notice that it is a vibrant and intense blue, more than in summer or spring.

It has this intense coloring because in autumn the Sun crosses the sky closer to the horizon; most of the sky is very angled to the Sun's rays, which reduces the red and green light levels, giving even more preference to the blue one.

The decrease in temperature also leads to a decrease in the humidity that accumulates in the sky, making it freer from the haze, which tends to spread all wavelengths.

Finally, to make this process even more evident, there is also another factor that concerns trees and leaves: compared to the green tones, the golden and orange tones typical of autumn contrast more visibly with the blue color, making it appear even more vivid.

Under such a wonderful sky it is not difficult to discover festive images, you must go a little further, inside the green that changes into gold and purple, inside the sap of the trees and dream. It is impossible to resist the beauty of a carefree dance of multicolored leaves. To sit on the benches and let yourself be covered by the soft foliage is something regenerating and beneficial. With imagination, believe me, you can do it whenever you want.

How wonderful it would be to be in the place of those spectacular leaves, to abandon yourself and let yourself be carried away by the wind, wherever he wants to push you, and find yourself there, immersed in this strange peace, in this flight to somewhere else. Amber leaves that vibrate in the air, that laugh, that chase each other fast. Devilish leaves that creep everywhere, lanceolate leaves that slip into your collar like so many small blades. Dreaming of falling on an immense mattress of crackling red leaves, sighing dead leaves. Turning their heads to cross their lost gaze, maybe they speak to people in a language that I do not understand, maybe they greet us, maybe they call us, maybe just mute, they fall. Use your imagination and they will use theirs for you, finding your connection.

Imagine the wind whistling and playing among the tallest branches of the trees, making the pine needles vibrate, caressing your face. Staring at the sky for a long time we will always find funny clouds chasing each other. Which of them will arrive first on the horizon? Some golden leaves remembered the blond hair of an angel, soft as a waterfall.

During so many enveloping and warm colors imagine you are a gnat in a plate of Indian turmeric, everything is red and grainy. The spice is fragrant, crunchy, slips and rolls under your thin paws.

The sand is soft, thin, as fine as powder, red as a peach pit, yellow, orange, ochre. It slips between your fingers, leaves its color on your fingertips, is soft underfoot, softer than any beach you have ever stepped on.

The pines cling to the overhangs, they protrude into the void to investigate the abyss, like imprudent children rocking on a balcony. They bump, they seem there to jump into the void. A tree, perhaps a birch tree, stands in the middle of the rocks, the red pinnacles, the pines with green needles: its leaves are yellow, they vibrate in the wind, they stand out against the green, red background of the landscape.

The drops of a recent rain have created on the red dust a complicated embroidery that is lost under the bushes, among the shrubs. What skilled lacemaker can create such a subtle and complicated weave? Small brown leaves are set inside, like sequins in a fabric.

Your orange fingers leave colored prints on the white paper. They look like the fingers of an Indian bride immersed in henna for an endless ceremony of lights, incense, and colors.

Above you are a large black crow with something in its beak. Birds are called and answered in many different languages from the silent corners of the forest. Scent of mushrooms, a memory of evenings around the table of the house in the mountains to clean the good mushrooms picked during the day's trip in the woods.

A tuft of heather is a stain of color at your feet, tiny flowers, tiny leaves that keep the old Ginkgo tree company. An old man and a little boy holding hands and weaving their roots under the ground.

Continue now to enjoy this precious opportunity to immerse yourself in the beauty of autumn. Imagine getting up slowly from the comfortable bench, adjust your pants and coat, take a deep breath, and you are on your way.

The park becomes more and more beautiful and colorful in its characteristic autumnal appearance.

Do you remember that fairy tale that was often told as children about the origins of autumn?

Why don't we remember it together?

A long time ago a large forest was populated by flowers, trees, animals, and goblins who played happily together, happy to enjoy the summer heat in the shade of the forest.

Walking among the trees it was also possible to hear some laughter of some irreverent elves who were not afraid to show themselves, but as the days went by the sun was always lower and lower on the horizon, and the heat was no longer so unbearable, the shadows got longer, and the darkness always came earlier.

Everyone in the forest knew that the time had come when one had to stop playing and playing around and start stocking up and getting ready for the long, cold winter.

The animals prepared their dens and food reserves for hibernation, the goblins collected wood and filled the pantries and the birds gathered to organize their long flight to the warm and food-rich lands of the south.

There was a lot of excitement, but every once in a while, someone would stop and think about summer and games, knowing that they were about to enter the cold season and would not be able to go out for a long time.

But there was someone who was hesitant for fear that the trees might get angry, they were always so serious, they controlled everything from the top of their branches, and it seemed that they never laughed...

But the enthusiasm of the goblin was not reduced, and he thought of coloring the trees at night, so that they would not notice anything.

So that night all the goblins climbed on the branches and colored the leaves of many colors: yellow, orange, red, brown, light, dark, and left some green. In the morning, when the sun illuminated the forest, the show was wonderful, even the trees were speechless.

The party was a great success, everyone in the forest got excited in front of that show of colors, laughed and sang all day until the evening when the goblins told the trees that they were ready to paint the leaves green as before.

It was the great chestnut tree, the old king of the forest, who asked the goblins to leave them so colorful, that they were beautiful and that they had never had so much fun as on that day, and that in any case the leaves would soon fall for the winter.

And so, every year since then, before winter steals the leaves from the trees, the goblins color them in these wonderful shades, a way to dress the great forest in a festive way!

Walking, it makes you want to play chase some pebbles between the leaves. There is no risk of hitting other passers-by and anyone can improvise as a footballer with a stone or a pinecone or a simple wood, or why not a big chestnut! I only suggest not to try to make two shots of foot with a chestnut hedgehog...!

Moving some leaves, some autumn flowers come to the fore. The flowers are not the exclusive prerogative of summer and spring, there are many types in autumn too. In particular, you can imagine noticing some beautiful purple flowers, and to recognize them even if you are not an expert, they are called "pansies of thought".

The meaning of the Pansy has always been linked to love, to the love between mother and daughter, to lovers, to those who do not want to be forgotten and who, by giving a Pansy as a gift, ask to think of him.

It is mythology that explains the meaning of the Pansy of thought.

It is said that Hades, god of the underworld, one day fell in love with Persephone, goddess of land and agriculture. Hades decided to marry Persephone and although Zeus agreed, Demeter, Persephone's mother, opposed the marriage. Hades then kidnapped the young girl while she was picking flowers and brought her to his kingdom. Demeter, desperate, wandered nine days and nine nights in search of the girl and the earth fell into desolation and frost: the plants died, and famine devastated the land, until Zeus sent Hermes, the messenger of the gods, to bring Persephone back to her mother. Zeus convinced Hades to an agreement: Persephone would spend four months in the Underworld and the rest of the year, between spring and autumn, would be with her mother. Demeter, appeased, returned to Mount Olympus and the earth was fertile and fertile again. While in the months when Persephone is in the underworld the earth is asleep and shrouded in winter. When at the beginning of spring Persephone returned for the first time among the living, the earth welcomed her and created for her new festive flowers, delicate and velvety like her eyes, true "thoughts of love" and invented the "pansies of thought". Since then, they have been returning on time every year, to celebrate Persephone, the goddess who represented the rebirth of nature in spring, who returns to earth.

According to the French population instead, it is said that in the petals you can see the face of your loved one, in France this flower is in fact called "pensée" and it is said that by looking at the petals of the flower you can see the face of your loved one.

Another legend tells of the mythological birth of the Pansy, created by Zeus to feed his beloved, transformed into a heifer.

It is a flower that sees its origins in Ethiopia, but also in South America, and that also sees it as native to New Zealand and Australia. Some people think that the Pansy is native to the Arab areas, since historically a very perfumed flower was widespread in those lands.

History teaches us that the violet was often used by the ancient Romans and Arabs as an addition to drinks to make them fragrant and more pleasant.

One last curiosity about this flower before going on: Pansy was a flower much loved by Napoleon Bonaparte. Perhaps the reason lies in the pleasant memory of the gesture made by his first wife, Josephine, who gave him a bouquet during their first date.

Go on your autumn walk some more, you are in no hurry to go anywhere.

You are not tired, you feel that the fresh air and a bit of movement are doing you good, refreshing body and soul.

You do not have any appointments scheduled.

You have no deadlines.

No one is waiting for you at home or in the store or in the office, you don't have to go to work, and everyone is safe and secure elsewhere while you can enjoy the sensational quiet that this autumn park is offering you.

Walking with carefreeness and eyes full of such beauty, you come across another good giant from the world of trees.

The American beech trees.

One of its strong points is the coloring of the foliage, alternate and ovate. The upper leaf, during the year, is dark green and shiny with small silvery hairs. It is autumn, so its leaves have quickly changed to a nice copper red and a bright yellow. The bark makes the beech interesting in all seasons; it is gray and smooth, with silvery reflections. Some people compare it to the skin of an elephant.

Another attraction are the fruits: beeches. In the shape of a hedgehog, they contain up to three small nuts. They have various alimentary uses, but they are precious especially because they become an unstoppable attraction for the fauna, nice and tender squirrels but especially birds.

To attract your attention this time, however, are neither the beautiful leaves nor the animals that populate its branches, but a beautiful little wooden house set among its strong and solid branches.

In the United States and in many parts of the world it is in fact a tree renowned for its strength and resistance to water, so much so that it was once used for the construction of ships.

There is a ladder inclined and well leaning against the trunk of the beech tree, it is very inviting.

The little house is splendid, built with a small entrance and some small windows, perfectly set between the branches.

Start slowly to climb the ladder. The steps are strong, there are no difficulties.

Arrived at the top of the house, you can enjoy the view from above. After a long walk you realize that the golden hour has arrived, the magical and most romantic hour of all: the hour of sunset.

Here you can admire the sky that turns a nice warm red, creating an atmosphere that reassures you, makes you feel protected, safe, that makes you forget every problem because the only thing you want to do is to watch the fantastic spectacle of the sunset. The clouds are lost on the horizon and with the last rays of the sun still present, you can already admire small bright dots in the sky, they are the first stars! And here on the opposite side appears the moon, the white lady, that just looking at her calms you, you understand that the evening has arrived and with it will come the night, synonymous of rest and bearer of advice. And it is beautiful to have your face lit by the last rays of the sun while everything around you seem to become magical.

The sun, the most bizarre artist in the universe, dyes the sky in various shades of pink, red, yellow, and orange as well as clouds and everything becomes a perfect picture.

The sunset can make us forget all the bad things that happened to us during the day because they are replaced by even more ancient and pleasant memories.

When the sensational spectacle of the sunset gives way to the noble night and its black mantle, the time comes for you to rest too.

After a long walk a restful sleep is what you need.

Then you enter the little wooden house, little by little.

Inside you will find a comfortable bed of leaves that the animals have prepared especially for you; they are very cozy with their human guests.

You snuggle on the leaves and discover that they are soft and comfortable, the scent of the forest and the earth that the night is raging with dew is very relaxing, there is no cold and there are no noises, except for the pleasant creaking of leaves.

And now it is time to rest your eyes, mind, and even your body.

Let go of the passing time and think only of the embrace of nature.

Let your body become one with nature.

You will sleep deeply, without any awakening that is not sweet and serene, because the trees protect you.

Take your time to find your favorite location, the important thing is that you are comfortable.

You are about to fall asleep deeply.

You will only dream of wise and ancient trees, colorful leaves and playful goblins, hedgehogs and squirrels, flowers, and ancient legends.

Enjoy the silence of the forest at night, the scents of wet earth, an ancestral contact with nature that welcomes you in its arms to accompany you in your sleep.

Let the embrace of leaves and trees accompany you in your sleep.

Sleep together with nature and the animals of the forest, in an ancient quietness that infuses peace and serenity.

The forest is asleep, everything rests now...

Chapter 2 Immerse Yourself in Relaxation

Welcome to another moment that must be dedicated entirely to yourself, your well-being and the care of your spirit and body.

First, take a deep, long breath, and just make yourself comfortable.

Prepare yourself entirely to receive positive vibrations, to relax, and above all let go of any bad thoughts and everything that weighs on your shoulders at this moment in your life.

Put something soft under your head, undress your shoes, unbuckle your belt if you are wearing one and do not keep clothes that tighten or make you feel uncomfortable. If it is evening, the best dress is a nice warm and enveloping pajama.

Let all the stress, anxiety and worries, or even depression, come out with your breath and let in the relief as you inhale.

Connect entirely with your state of detachment from reality, let yourself be transported elsewhere, to a dimension where you are the center of everything, where every creature is busy pampering you and loving you.

There are only people smiling and without ulterior motives around you, there is no falsehood but only love, peace, and serenity.

Everything is designed so that you feel welcomed and safe.

You are safe here, protected and loved.

The atmosphere is relaxing and welcoming, the environment is full of colors that make you feel good, that you like, that are your favorite.

You can hear laughter and cheerfulness not far from you.

You are surrounded by affection and love; everyone is here just for you.

You have nothing to keep under control here, you do not have to think about anything, there is no deadline, no clocks, no phones, or agenda.

You must feel like your only main commitment is to breathe, inhale and exhale, relax, and enjoy the peace and quiet of the moment.

Now imagine you are in an environment like a spa, in a magnificent massage center, where the walls have soft colors, and the lights are soft, and many candles are lit here and there.

Stress is the great enemy of modern times. We all lead fast-paced lives, we have to manage a multitude of deadlines and at work we feel more and more the pressure to keep up performance and not disappoint anyone, so you don't have to feel lonely, we are all in the same boat. Stress affects many people at work every year. But we are here together to get rid of this common enemy and you have already managed to get rid of it by taking this moment of relaxation for yourself.

There are various ways to vent stress, such as doing sports, but to prevent it from arising in the future you need a more reasoned approach, that's why to make you relax with a story I thought for you a relaxing massage with candles.

Most massages, regardless of the type, has among its benefits that of giving relaxation to the body.

In this story I thought for you a relaxing massage that focuses solely on the relaxing effect, which is the reason why it is done, thus being more effective than other types for this purpose.

Among the benefits of relaxation massage, there is a reduction in blood pressure, anxiety, and stress levels. The relaxation massage stimulates the production of endorphins, thus improving the mood of those who receive it.

Of course, ours will be an imaginary massage, but if you concentrate and let go totally for your mind it will be like having received it.

You are here for a precious treatment that takes place as a real sensory ritual, you are going to enjoy a long and beneficial relaxing massage.

Imagine you are already lying on your stomach on a comfortable bed, with some soft warm cotton towels to cover you.

You are perfectly at ease.

This massage is a relaxing massage, but we can count it among the rituals of wellness, it has its origins in Ayurveda, for which body and mind are closely related. So, the massage will relax your mind for a complete well-being that also involves your spirit!

The warm candlelight, the vegetable butter that melts slowly and turns into oil and slowly with the touch of hands and forearms slides over the body. A sweet whirl of fragrances and pleasant emotions that delight the senses.

A multi-sensory journey that will immerse you in complete relaxation and abandonment of the senses.

The relaxing power of the colors of candlelight blends with the feeling of harmony and balance transmitted by the heady scents of essential oils.

Imagine that there are also oriental melodies in the background during the massage, certain sounds like a flute, or a flowing stream, or Tibetan bells, represent an additional ally against stress, thanks to the beneficial effects of music therapy.

Let yourself be pampered by the pleasant sensation of drops, of the light and fluid vegetable butter that arrives on your skin with a gentle heat, dissolving tensions, giving pleasure, restoring tone and vigor to the body, freeing it from inhibitions and fatigue, recharging it with well-being and new passions.

The massage, widely understood, is a real pampering for everyone. It brings with it a renewed state of well-being, but when it comes to relaxing massage, this panacea condition, balance, and recovery of one's inner energy is accentuated even more.

The use of massage, to eliminate fatigue, relieve pain, relax, and allow easier application of oils and ointments on the skin, is lost in the mists of time.

Probably, it represents the oldest form of medical treatment.

The first historical references related to it date back as far as two thousand seven hundred B.C. and are present in some documents from Ancient China and India. From then to the present day this technique has spread like wildfire, gradually taking on different characteristics depending on the various cultures of the peoples who treasured it.

Other references to massage are also in texts of Indian medicine, always very ancient.

Hieroglyphics testify that from India these notions moved to Mesopotamia and Egypt, but also to Greece, thanks to Alexander the Great who conquered some Indian territories.

It is well known for example that the Egyptians in Cleopatra's time loved to be massaged immersed in pools of scented water.

Many other ancient cultures such as the Maya, Hawaiian, Inca, Navajo, and Cherokee cultures, for example, used massage as a healing technique against diseases and as a means of prevention.

Even the poet Homer and the doctor Hippocrates were convinced supporters of massage and exalted its therapeutic virtues.

The Greeks developed various massage techniques, the most important of which were sports massage, games massage and healing massage.

The massage also moved to Italy, in ancient Rome.

Here it was practiced at first in spas, later also as a sports massage for gladiators.

It is said that Julius Caesar used to get massaged every day to find relief from the pain of migraine and neuralgia due to epilepsy while Celsius, a Roman doctor, was convinced that you should massage your body several times a day, possibly in the open air using the sun.

The Greek doctor Galen also devoted much of his time to writing several texts about massage techniques.

In the Olympic Games held in honor of Zeus in Olympia, athletes were awarded with oil amphorae and the winner was crowned with olive branches, but above all it was common custom among athletes to massage the body with olive oil.

However, the cult of massage was interrupted during the Middle Ages, because of the obscurantism that considered it sinful and was rediscovered only in the Renaissance period.

The development and evolution of massage lasted thousands of years until advances in modern medicine and technology were able to set aside what was the first form of treatment until the Twentieth Century.

The relaxing massage has the function of stimulating relaxation starting from awareness.

Awareness of your body, your feelings, your emotions. Here is what this practice intervenes in.

The relaxing massage is much more than a treatment that relieves stress. The benefits that it can bring are fantastic, of great scope and go to interest both body and spirit. It helps to overcome the phenomena of insomnia caused by psychological tension and stress and helps to actively intervene on the body.

Following a holistic approach, the relaxing massage has the function of rebalancing the seven chakras, the energy meridians, the flows, to allow you to find what we all have always wanted: balance and lost energy.

Research and several studies have shown that relaxing massage therapies, especially when combined with complementary treatments such as soft light and candles, relaxing music, pleasant oils and scents, can help to significantly reduce symptoms such as anxiety, tension, agitation and frustration.

These can provide deep relaxation and relieve some of the psychological aspects of stress.

Here are some benefits related to this treatment:

Reduction of stress and anxiety.
Improved sleep quality.

Reduction of agitation.

Containment of anxiety-related behavioral problems.

Promotion of relaxation of the whole body.

Stimulation of circulation.

Ability to give comfort to the whole body.

Reduction of pain threshold.

Decrease in muscle stiffness.

Ability to regenerate the body by providing balance, calm and well-being.

An anti-stress treatment, as can also be simply the descriptive listening to images, contexts and relaxing actions, a story like the one you are listening to fall asleep better and deeply, which leads your mind to focus on something beneficial and positive, does not only act in contrast to all the possible consequences to which tension, haste, depression and anxiety can lead. There is more, much more. This treatment also helps to increase willpower, tenacity, and optimism.

All the movements performed during a relaxing massage are dictated by the most intimate sensuality. The circular movements bring to the surface the most beautiful and instinctive sensations that stress and daily worries suffocate it is on these that one must concentrate during the massage. The anti-stress massage reconnects mind, body, and soul, bringing them back into the present moment, removing fears and distractions.

One of the most extensive and typical effects of anti-stress massage is the ability to bring back the person who undergoes the massage to their primordial condition of well-being and balance.

This practice is linked to the energy and the flow of sensations, emotions, passions that in our existence find their atavistic, primordial, and innate source of life.

One of the most extensive and typical effects of anti-stress massage is the ability to bring back the person who undergoes the massage to their primordial condition of well-being and balance.

This practice is linked to the energy and the flow of sensations, emotions, passions that in our existence find their atavistic, primordial, and innate source of life.

So, the anti-stress massage makes a happy entrance in our everyday life, giving us a great possibility: to find harmony, peace, relaxation, therefore, a definitive solution to all the problems that come from stress.

It is, as you can well understand, a unique experience of its kind, a complete sensory experience, which, as such, brings to light, with extraordinarily synchronic concomitance, feelings and sensations that we carry within us since our birth. Immerse yourself in the massage means living, on your skin - in this case really in every sense - what can be considered, with good reason, a real mood therapy ... the therapy of physical, emotional, and psychological well-being.

You just must imagine and relax completely.

Imagine now that there is someone, a man or a woman doesn't matter at all, just think that it is a trusted person who wants to take loving care of you by giving you a relaxing massage.

Just know that from now on we will call him the masseur, a person dressed entirely in white.

White symbolizes spirituality, it is the color of angels. White is associated with purity and wisdom, it emanates a lively, clear, and fresh energy.

White contains the vibrations of peace, love, and calm. White is the color of those who give and spread light. On the contrary, the energy of black takes from what is around and absorbs light.

Let us start with a foot massage.

Feel that the massage starts at the sole of the foot, compressed with both hands, the masseur first rubs the top and then the sole and here begins to perform movements going up to the top, gradually decreasing the intensity of the foot massage. Then massage the heel.

Draw small circles virtually: apply firm pressure in this area. After the entire heel, continue rubbing both thumbs up and down. While one thumb moves up, the other one goes down.

Then massage the ankles. Again, imagine you feel circular movements using both hands, one on the inside and the other on the outside.

Feel it then gently rub the bone itself, applying pressure with your knuckles on this area. Rotate the wrist back and forth massaging very gently. Massage your toes as well. Massage gently and slowly first, and faster later.

At this point the masseur starts to sprinkle oil on the legs, starting from the tip of the foot, with circular movements from the bottom up to the hips.

Today we have lost contact with our body. It is good to rediscover it: to do so, we start with a relaxing leg massage. By bringing energy back to the legs and feet, our body is helped to release blocked tension and encourage more natural, slender, and energetic movements.

So, imagine that the masseur now lovingly continues towards your back.

The sense of touch is a unique, unequivocal sensation that comforts, envelops, relaxes, and stimulates like nothing in the world. The massage produces positive effects for both those who do it and those who receive it.

The relaxing back massage begins by treating the lumbar area with light, circular movements, varying in intensity and pressure. The movements, fluid but firm, serve to warm the skin and relax the muscles. The masseur then moves on to perform touching movements, starting to exert more and more pressure as the treatment progresses.

After these touches, the masseur opens your hands in a fan-shaped manner by sliding your hands along the sides of your body, following, always with your hands, all the shapes of your body, pressing, in particular, on the muscles on both sides of your spine, then sliding them slowly and enveloping along your hips.

Afterwards, proceed in reverse, going up from your back to your shoulders, always massaging firmly upwards with one hand while the other goes down along your hips. The massage movement should always be rhythmic and well controlled, so that it is pleasant and fluid.

The tension in the back is relieved, the cellular memory is awakened from its torpor. Emotions flow smoothly. Where there was pain there is relaxation, where there is detachment there is empathy.

The touch of the skin has a great importance: it acts as a caress, a pampering, but it also serves to restore balance, serenity, tapping into the depths of the body and psyche. The relaxing back massage also benefits the psyche. The contact of the hands on the epidermis transmits a message of sensuality, reciprocity, passion, and deep trust to the brain.

The massage continues, and now as expected the masseur moves towards the neck and head.

The relaxing head massage starts from the centrality that this delicate part of the body has in our body. It is one of the most mysterious, most fascinating, privileged seats not only of the five senses, but also the center that houses the brain, with its millions of endings. If performed correctly, the massage of the head is equivalent to a full-body massage.

In the process of fetal development, the brain is the first organ that is formed. At birth it is larger and heavier than any other organ. Therefore, head massage has a very central role in the healing therapy that passes from body massage.

Head massage has its origins in Indian treatments based on the ancient Ayurvedic form of healing that dates back almost 4,000 years. This formula acts, according to tradition, on the three superior chakras: Vishuddha, Ajna and Sahasrara. This relaxing treatment, in fact, in addition to being a real panacea, can ensure a serene harmony that will be reflected throughout the body.

Now the masseur dedicates himself to the base of the head. First placing one hand at the base of your neck and the other gently on your forehead.

The masseur will then proceed with opening the hand on the neck by sliding it over the back until it reaches the vertebrae: here, he exerts a slight pressure. The relaxing neck massage then goes up to the vertebrae, from the vertebrae up to the hairline: stay there for a moment exerting light pressure and then repeat the movement.

All movements are soft and are performed with extreme caution and slowly.

The relaxing head and neck massage help to soothe insomnia as few natural treatments in the world can do.

As a final touch of pampering and relaxation, the masseur will take care of your hands.

Many are accustomed to considering the hands as an organ capable of doing, giving, and taking objects and things. They allow you to take and leave, build materially, put together and separate, approach or move away.

The palm of the hand has the largest amount per surface area of tactile receptors and is therefore defined as the seat of touch. Thanks to this extreme receptive sensitivity the hand can also be considered as an organ capable of receiving stimuli that, in turn, can, by reflected communication, transmit to apparatuses and organs as well.

To proceed with the hand massage, the masseur makes delicate and intense movements at the same time, starting from the area of the wrists to the phalanges. Then he imagines receiving soft movements especially along the palm of the hand and does the same for all the fingers.

First one hand, then the other.

The massage is finished, and the masseur covers you with an incredibly soft warm cotton towel.

The bed on which you have been lovingly massaged and relaxed has become wonderfully comfortable, and gradually the curtains are closing, and the lights are dimming more and more. The music is now a light background sound. With a light breath the candles are blown out one by one, and in the air expands with fragrances that smell of exotic and distant worlds.

Only a small incense remains lit, a wooden stick that will incinerate itself.

They are olfactory notes and chords that by their nature favor the openness of the mind and generate a feeling of peace.

First, the incense, in all its declensions, with all the meaning of purification that it brings with it according to the various cultures. And then the balsamic resins, the woody notes of sandalwood and vetiver, iris. The scents that remind us of the pure air from a mountain peak to the solitary walks in the early morning rain. But also, the simple vanilla, which not only makes anyone feel at ease instantly, but has calming properties and can help you find sleep faster.

And finally, lavender, A study published in a leading scientific journal reveals that lavender oil acts on the brain by increasing sleepiness. Imagine you could choose the fragrance in you would rather be wrapped before sleep.

Now try to take advantage of this state of deep calm. As the worries go away, the silence of the nerve cells discovers at the occasion of this moment of well-being, our true personality.

Follow the amount and rhythm of your breathing, passively.

Having just finished a relaxing massage it will be normal for you to feel a little tired, slightly numb, even a little sore, all this is completely normal; we must not forget that these are the reactions due to the activation of the body, which is called, precisely through the massage, to regain lost balance.

You are completely relaxed now and ready to let it all go.

Everyone has taken care of you, loved you, massaged and pampered you.

You feel great.

Whenever you want you will always find someone ready to prepare for you a massage room with the colors you prefer, with covering curtains so that no one can peek inside and see what happens, with lighted candles that spread a flickering light, warm, romantic and enveloping.

In the air you can imagine smelling your favorite scents, maybe sun creams or hay, which will take you back to places of childhood or simply when you were traveling in a seaside resort.

If you feel the need, all you have to do is make yourself comfortable and at ease and you will know how to find the perfect balance between body and mind, balancing the relaxation between limbs and thoughts, so that everything is catalyzed by the relaxing massage.

The relaxing massage also involves a sense of emotional liberation, no less important, especially in view of the hectic and stressful rhythm that characterizes the life of us all.

You have released the tension and relaxed the mind and body.

You have found relief, energy, and psychophysical well-being.

Now you just must enjoy this relaxing environment to allow yourself a long sleep, which after a relaxing massage will be deep and regenerating.
Close your eyes and listen only to your breath, let yourself go to the dreams that are coming.

Relax and let sleep massage you along with your dreams.

It will be a night of serenity and renewed awareness.

Have a good sleep.

Chapter 3 Animal Love

Hi, here we are together again. How are you?

Are you ready to enjoy another moment dedicated to reaching together a place or a feeling of peace and self-respect?

As usual, it is important that you make yourself comfortable and at ease.

There should be no noise or distractions around you, as much as you can make sure you isolate yourself and find a private corner where no one will come to disturb you.

Are you settled well? Are you sitting in a soft armchair with a warm blanket on your legs or have you already brushed your teeth and slipped into bed with pajama?

Don't worry about looking inadequate. I will try to guess, you are afraid of appearing too aged or a bit "loser", aren't you? Please, do not joke! All of us, even the powerful or famous people, your idols of reference or those you consider cool and strong, sometimes need to sit in an armchair like old people or to be put to bed with the blankets tucked up properly.

Don't you believe it?

Well, it makes no difference. If that is what you really need, then do it!

Do you know that a good night's sleep will make you feel better, right? Well, that is why then you must indulge your spirit and your body and prepare them the way to fall asleep with ease and gentleness. If this involves going to bed early, or sitting in your grandmother's armchair, then do not hesitate!

Ok, now that you are in the mood, we are ready to dive into a fantastic world full of love and pure hearts.

What am I talking about?

Angels with tails.

That is to say: dogs, cats, horses, rabbits, donkeys, and the whole wonderful world of animals.

It doesn't matter that you already have a pet in your house, if you have one you will surely already know what I'm talking about, but if you don't have one then let yourself be carried away by this story in an enchanted place where you can pet, chase, play and get some licked by a four-legged friend.

Scientific studies have proven that a complex and delicate harmony is established between a domestic animal and a human being that stimulates emotional triggering and promotes openness to new experiences, new ways of communicating, new interests.

The animal does not judge, does not refuse, gives itself totally, stimulates smiles, helps socialization, increases self-esteem and above all has no form of prejudice towards others.

Animals are good for health.

In the presence of discomfort, they are an incredibly powerful support with obvious effects on well-being.

Several studies have shown that during an encounter with an animal, anxiety is reduced.

Even for those who suffer from depression, contact with an animal is stimulating.

Of course, you'll be comfortable in your position all the time, but if you let your imagination run wild and put aside any form of resistance you'll see that it will be exactly like having taken a ride in a riding stable with lots of horses, in a place with some puppies of dog or cat and why not give a carrot to a nice donkey.

In modern society where people live surrounded by technology, blue lights, applications, and social networks, it becomes even more essential and fundamental for people to maintain contact with nature and exchange with another living being. For example, the encounter with an animal enriches the person in many ways: reinforcing the ability to stay in the present - because animals treasure the past but do not ask questions about their future as we all constantly do - and to be open to the outside world, recovering or discovering their own instinct, developing the sharing and respect for the needs of the other.

Letting go and being pampered by an animal helps us to overcome traumas and fears, improving self-knowledge.

Imagine being on a beautiful farm like the ones you see in the movies, with all the stereotypes typical of the case, all made of wood, with the flag of the nation flying and swaying moved by the wind, tall beech and oak trees in the surroundings, spruce trees, and endless expanses of fields. Outside is parked a red off-road vehicle dirty with mud and earth, as it must be, and a huge tractor is parked next to the hay sheaves.

A beautiful puppy runs up to you, a dog with a sweet and mild look, who wags his tail cheerfully and happily and has a mad desire to lick your whole face.

It doesn't matter what breed of dog you have, it can also be a nice half-breed, or it can be like the one you had as a child or, why not, the dog you saw in the park and that particularly attracted your attention.

"The dog is man's best friend". How many times have we heard this sentence? Infinite times, so much so that we no longer grasp its true meaning. When you think about it, however, it is not a stereotype: among all our "cousins" of the animal kingdom, the dog is the one with whom we manage to establish the most intense relationship, the deepest and longest lasting emotional exchange.

You know, our furry friends are able to give affection spontaneously and sincerely, without any prejudice, conditioning or falsification - a characteristic that all animals have in common, distinguishing them from humans, but which is particularly accentuated in dogs. No psychological defensive mechanism, calculation, or interest comes into play in them when they decide to establish an emotional relationship with us.

In addition, dogs can read human body language and to perceive the emotional state through its hormonal secretions: anxiety or worry, fear or sadness. It does not end there: perceived an emotion in the subject, dogs react with liveliness, play, physical contact, cuddles, and warmth.

Would you like to caress him?

We too, through our caresses and manipulations, can communicate with the dog by transferring clear and explicit messages.

Petting a dog along the cheek, under the chin, chest and side is a sign of great attention and respect that keeps the dog calm, receptive to the pleasure of these caresses, on the contrary, caressing a dog on the head, between the ears, neck and rump communicates a certain degree of authority and dominance that not all dogs are willing to accept.

Do you know that dogs talk to us? And you will ask yourself: how to understand them?

Dogs are highly intelligent animals and have developed different techniques to "talk to them". You only need to recognize the signals...

They will not use words or text messages, but dogs do talk to us, you just need to know how to understand them.

Our four-legged friends, in fact, are intelligent animals and during their evolution have developed a language all their own performed with precise body movements.

How to understand what the cute puppy on the farm is telling you?

Know that when a dog wags its tail it means that it is happy or excited, but the dog's tail can represent different moods. For example, when it is straight and perpendicular to the body, it means that our friend is intrigued by something, maybe some animal spotted in the distance, while if it is upright above the head, it expresses aggression.

When instead the tail is low and gathered between the legs (the famous "tail between the legs") it means that the dog is scared!

Are you not convinced that while you are bending over to give and receive the cuddles and parties from a nice puppy dog this creature is talking to you?

Then, perhaps reconciling perhaps even more sleep, let me tell you a few stories about it.

Once upon a time there was a lady who went with a friend in search of mushrooms to make many wonderful recipes with this special ingredient, but unfortunately, she is stung by a wasp. The lady, allergic, is quickly taken by anaphylactic shock, is no longer breathing and panics. The friend calls immediately to activate the rescue, but the rescue is slow to arrive because the two women have entered a dense forest and it is difficult to locate them. And so, Sheila, the faithful dog of the friend who was with them, instead of staying there as the canine instinct would command, to lick the dying woman's hand, starts like a rocket, without hesitation and with great courage, crosses the woods, finds the rescuers and guides them skillfully in the right place saving the life of the lady.

This is a true story. In a case like this we are not faced with a simple instinctive behavior; we are faced with an "intelligent" behavior, in which the dog does not respond to the command of instinct (do not move away from the wounded) but elaborates "a complex plan including the involvement of other individuals".

This story suggests a very ancient and vast literature concerning the reasoning skills of dogs. One of the texts that has most influenced posterity is the "Natural History" of Pliny, which deals with the voice of fish and birds, but spreads widely on canine intelligence, cites a dog who had recognized in the crowd the killer of his master and with his bites and barking had forced him to confess the crime, or the dog of a condemned man on death row howling sadly, when a spectator had thrown food at him, he approached the dead man's mouth, and when the corpse had been thrown into the river he had swam, in an attempt to support him.

But the most philosophically interesting discussion on canine intercourse had already developed for at least three centuries in a debate between Stoics, academics, and Epicureans (Epicureans were philosophical followers of Epicurus and believed that happiness was the supreme good of life and that virtue consists in the liberation of disturbance).

In the context of the stoic discussion appears a topic attributed to Crisippus, that will be resumed and popularized almost five centuries later by Sixth Empiricus. Sixth believed that the dog was able to execute a perfect logical reasoning, proof was that a dog, arrived at a crossroads, and having recognized with the smell that the prey has not taken two of the roads, it rushes immediately for the third without even sniffing. In fact, the dog would somehow do this reasoning: "The prey either took this way or that, or the other; now it is neither this one nor that one; and therefore, it is the other" (which would be an example of a reasoning).

Sixth also remembered that the dog possesses a "logos" because he knows how to remove splinters and wipe away sores, keeps the sick limb immobile, and identifies herbs that can soothe his suffering. As for an animal language, it is true that we do not understand the voices of animals, but neither do we understand the voices of colors whose idiom is unknown to us, which yet speak; and dogs certainly emit different voices in different situations.

In Plutarch's "De sollertia animalium" it is said that certainly animal rationality is imperfect compared to human rationality, but these differences also exist between human beings.

In one of his writings Elian, in addition to the arguments already seen, mentions dogs that fall in love with human beings.

In "De abstinentia" by Porfirio the arguments in favor of animal intelligence serve to support a "vegetarian" thesis.

All topics that will be variously taken up in modern times and up to the present day.

But let us stop here: even if it is not possible to define canine intelligence well, we should be more sensitive to this mystery and get in relation with the purity that defines the animal soul.

Let me just leave you an interesting fact: in the thirteenth century, the Mongolian emperor Kublai Khan owned as many as five thousand Tibetan mastiffs that he used for hunting and war. Just think, never in the course of history has such many animals belonging to one person been equaled. The kennel of Kublai Khan, according to legends, had to be of considerable size to contain the thousands of Tibetan mastiffs, one of the largest breeds in the world. Beyond the use of the emperor and its imposing size, the Tibetan mastiff is a dog with a docile and gentle nature.

Imagine now, after having cuddled and interacted for a long time with the cute and playful puppy dog, to be attracted by a beautiful cat meowing in your direction.

The kitten is half lying on the low branch of a tree and seems to want to receive some loving caresses.

Some of us prefer to approach dogs, which are much more open and welcoming, or simple so to speak, than cats, but if you can connect with a cat it is something unique and exceptional.

It is important to meet the cat calmly, without imposing too narrow distances and wait for him to welcome us.

In this sense, it is also important to avoid abrupt movements and loud noises that could frighten the animal and take you away from winning the cat's confidence. The cats, in fact, do not like people too agitated and noisy, so when you are in their presence it is necessary to speak in a calm and quiet voice in order to create a relaxed environment, where the cat can feel comfortable and free to interact with its surroundings respecting its time.

You must also remember that looking into the eyes of a kitten is interpreted as a provocative attitude. So, to win the cat's confidence, keep him calm and tell him that you do not want to hurt him, you can look at him, but without staring too long. After all, since childhood we have been taught that it is not good manners to stare too long at someone, right?

Now think about sitting next to this tree and waiting for the cat to take its first steps towards you.

Slowly, with slow, sinuous movements, without making any noise, the cat comes closer, reaches you and even comes to rub against your legs, but be careful, this does not necessarily mean that it is giving you permission to touch it.

You can therefore do a little test to assess her predisposition towards you: offer her the tip of your index finger to sniff, with the rest of her hand closed with your fist. On average, a cat cannot resist this gesture and, if well disposed, will not be limited to a sniff, but will go further by rubbing the chubby cheeks against your finger, raising the chin and inviting you to scratch right there. In practice it will be the cat himself to suggest how to caress it, perhaps going so far as to rub the back of the neck against the palm of your hand, inciting you to purr, with his eyes ajar. And this is exactly what happens with the cat of our imaginary farm.

Under the chin, behind the ears and at the back at the base of the tail: these are some of the places where cats usually prefer to receive caresses and scratches.

Imaginarily he starts to run his hand along his hair starting from the head, between the ears, starting with a scratch, and then continue with a light caress that follows the curves of his back, to get down to the base of the tail, where most likely the very enjoyable feline will like another scratch.

Cats have calming effects on our body: they help to reduce anxiety, stress and insomnia problems, they also help to improve your self-esteem, your sociality with others. The purring of the cat is one of the most perceptible and beneficial stimuli that anyone can immediately notice.

The cat, while being a reserved and solitary animal, can also be a little egocentric enough to adapt well to the role of the protagonist of many popular legends around the world.

I will tell you some of them:

On Noah's Ark during the Universal Flood, mice were reproducing very quickly, putting the survival of other animals at risk. Noah did not know how to solve the problem and turned to the Lord for help. Here the lion sneezed and from his sneeze two cats were born and they were able to bring the number of mice back to an acceptable level.

The Persian army, commanded by Cambyses, besieged Pelusius, finding the resistance of the Egyptian army. Unable to defeat the Egyptian guard, Cambyses decided to have his army capture as many live cats as possible. After three days the Persian army launched a new attack using the cats as a shield. The Egyptians, in order not to hurt the cats in the fight, decided to surrender.

In a Japanese legend it is said that in Tokyo lived an old lady so poor that she was even forced to sell her cat. Sometime later the cat appeared to her in a dream, asking her to create a statue of her with clay. The lady made the statuette that she was able to sell. The success was so great that the old lady became rich because she invented this statuette, the Maneki Neku, the famous cat who welcomes with his paw up.

From a Finnish legend we can learn that there is a place in Finland, a place where it is very cold, where it is said that a witch can suddenly arrive in the house and with a spell brings everyone present on a sleigh pulled by a huge cat accompanying them into the world of night and evil spirits.

In a Polish legend it is said that a cat grieved because her master had thrown her cats in the river continued to meow desperately. The willows on the long river, in pity, stretched the branches towards the water to allow the little kittens to cling and save themselves. Since that moment in Spring the willows have not bloomed but as a reminder of this event, they are covered with inflorescences covered with soft fluff like the coat of a kitten.

Finally, it is written in a European legend that the inhabitants of a village, in order to get help in building a bridge, made a pact with the devil, promising him in exchange for help the soul of the first being who had crossed the bridge. On the day of the inauguration, the bishop convinced a black cat to cross the bridge thus saving the soul of his faithful and mocking the devil.

D. Defoe's novel "Robinson Crusoe" is inspired by the experiences of the Scottish sailor Alexander Selkirk. In the early eighteenth century the sailor found himself abandoned on an island off the coast of Chile. He enjoyed the company of cats on the island who had survived previous shipwrecks. The cats became his friends for over four and a half years on the island, helping him to keep his nerve in the face of total solitude and the threat of cannibals.

An ancient French legend tells of the existence of a stray cat, the Matagot, which brings luck and is looking for a master. To win his favor, it is necessary to offer him roast chicken as a meal and then invite him into the house. The first night the Matagot is in the house, he must have the food from the same dish as the owner. As a reward, the Matagot will give the human being gold coins and lots of luck.

I hope these short legends have made you smile, because I have another fictional tale in store for you from Anglo-Saxon folklore.

What is the origin of the purr? Haven't you ever asked yourself that?

If I have guessed, then let us discover this story together.

Once upon a time there was a king and his queen who, after a long time and numerous attempts, finally managed to have a daughter. Overwhelmed with joy, when a gypsy offered to read the future of the newborn, they accepted with enthusiasm... enthusiasm that became despondency when this gypsy announced to them with a serious air that if the princess had ever offered herself in marriage to a prince, she would fall victim to a fatal disease.

Under the advice of the gypsy, three white cats were placed as guardians of the princess' health.

At the disposal of the felines were placed as much flaxen balls as gold balls: if the princess was safe, the three cats would play with only flaxen balls. If, instead, her life had been in danger, they would have paid attention to the golden balls.

Everything went well for the first years of the princess' life. One day, however, a few years later, a charming prince with a noble soul showed up at court; the girl tried until the last moment to reject her feelings, but in the end prince and princess confessed their feelings to each other.

And the three feline guardians started playing with golden balls.

Soon, the gypsy's prophecy was fulfilled...with one variation: it was not the princess who fell ill, but the prince. Within twenty-seven days her life was destined to be extinguished unless the princess was able to weave ten thousand skeins of linen without help from other hands.

It was an impossible task, and the princess was aware of it. But just when it seemed that all was lost, her three white cats spoke to her for the first time and offered her their help. "Ours are paws, not hands," they said, "and therefore we can go away with you".

So, the princess and her cats worked hard. Together, with dedication, love and will power, they managed to save the prince's life.

After the happy success and the happy ending, as a reward for their devotion and generosity, the cats received as a gift the jewels of the princess they loved to play with... and the ability to purr.

According to British folklore, this is how the cats started purring. But of course, there are many other legends.

Have you enjoyed enough of the farm cat's incredibly special purring?

Here you are immediately attracted by a nitrite, yes, because there is a beautiful horse waiting for you in its enclosure.

Imagine entering the barn, immediately you are overwhelmed by an extraordinarily strong smell of barn, it is a pungent and pungent smell, heavy and almost intolerable, but also has something surprisingly familiar. The smell of the stable immediately sends our memory back to farms, scenes of life in the countryside, moments of serenity and quiet, quiet days in which time is marked only by the natural rhythm of the countryside, the sun and the needs of the animals.

Moreover, for horses, cows and donkeys and other stable animals their smell is fundamental.

Let me tell you about the importance of barn smell, so that you, even in your imagination, can bear it better.

In times gone by, the horse was linked to the possibility to make movements for public or private commitments, when public services were not available. Horses were tied to gigs or carriages to transport people but also goods, and often the routes were quite fixed and repetitive, and it was said that the horse, after having retraced the same route for many years, knew the road by heart.

It was above all in the return that the horse did not need guidance or particulars commands, because, it was said, when he approached home, he "smelled the barn". In this regard, many concrete cases were cited that proved that the horse had this sense of recognition of its stable.

Now that we have entered the stable, you are in front of this noble, proud, and majestic animal, a dream for many children, but also for adults.

It takes a lot of time and patience, however, to learn how to approach a horse.

You can imagine it in a beautiful chocolate brown color, tending to fawn, or white as in fairy tales, or spotted, in short, it may be the type of horse that you would like to meet.

The first time we approach a horse we usually tend to want to caress its snout, well, there is nothing more wrong. The snout is an overly sensitive part for the horse and extremely intimate. You can only get close to this part of the body when you have become familiar with the horse.

As I said, it takes time and patience to gain his confidence. First, it is necessary to give him as much space as possible, letting him approach us in his own time. It is wrong to approach him, but it is also wrong to ignore him.

The situation is unblocked when the horse will move towards us, showing interest. At this point it is essential to remain calm and avoid making sudden movements that could agitate the horse, which is sensitive and can perceive the mood of the people around it. Once you have established a bond with the horse you can start pampering him lovingly.

The caress is an affectionate gesture, but even in the best intentions the reactions are different depending on the points of the body that we are going to caress. In the case of the horse the most suitable caress, the one that reassures and pleases him, is the one on the rump, neck or withers, the part between the mane and shoulder blades. Once a certain bond of trust has been established with this special creature, it will also be possible to position yourself in front of him, caressing his snout between his eyes.

This point is very delicate, and it is recommended to approach it only when we are sure that the horse already trusts us. The caress should always be light, delicate, and never abrupt or reckless, because a wrong movement can frighten him and bring the contact path back to the starting point.

Come to think about it, we should also adopt this behavior among ourselves, from one human being to another. But above all, with ourselves.

Moreover, before starting to caress the horse it is always good to let him hear his own voice, speaking to him in a calm and at the same time safe way. The horse must always perceive our tranquility, that is why even if with imagination I wanted to take you to visit and get to know a horse.

Hey, who is behind the horse fence?

A genuinely nice and cheerful little donkey!

With donkeys, however, the situation is slightly different, but also with them we must spend time and patience to gain trust and mutual affection. However, it is a firmer animal than the horse, which infuses a sense of greater reflexivity and calm. It has even been discovered that the donkey induces a lot of self-telling, perhaps because it can be taken on a walk, in the paddock or in a park or in a forest and have a chat with it. Yes, a chat with a donkey, what is wrong with that? How many of us talk to the family dog or cat? Almost everyone who has one at home. And it comes to us normal! So why not also talk to the donkey? If we are depressed or stressed while we are on the subway to get to work or we are anxious for an interview or a meeting, we could think of that time in a story someone suggested we imagine a farm and have a chat with a donkey during a walk. Uh, I almost forgot unlike the horse, the donkey has unbelievably soft hair and a strong feeling of calm.

Hoping that the tour of the farm has conveyed the serenity, peace and harmony that reigns in the hearts of our animal friends, I tell you one last moral about them through small anecdotes.

Some time ago I saw a very moving video on the net, on a busy ring road of a metropolitan city, a dog tries to cross the street and is hit by a car. As a result of the collision, he loses consciousness and lies unconscious on the ground, grazed by dozens of cars coming up non-stop. Another dog, putting his life at risk, ventures onto the same road and with enormous effort manages to drag what is perhaps one of his pack mates to the side of the road, where shortly afterwards humans intervene to help him.

How can you explain the behavior of the second dog? Why did he risk his life to save another's? If we wanted to draw a quick conclusion, it could only be this: the dog acted morally, showing compassion for his companion, and behaving accordingly, despite the enormous danger he had to face. Also note how the dog did not, as usually happens, drag the other dog by the scruff of the neck, but moved him more gently - and laboriously - wrapping him with his front paws.

Well, this is certainly not the only case. Elephants have been caught trying to push and support the matriarch of the herd to continue the march despite its obvious difficulty, female gorillas have been sighted saving unfortunate children in their cage, and I could add many other similar events.

All these examples, which are obviously only a small sample, seem to demonstrate one thing only: animals can act in a moral way, showing compassion for their fellow humans and deciding in some cases to sacrifice their own selfish interests.

Perhaps, the whole of humanity, by reconciling with the animal kingdom, could heal many of the ugliness that have plagued society for centuries, and in particular modern sociality.

In the meantime, we will always know where we can give and receive a caress without fear of being misunderstood, judged, or rejected.

A wet nose, a soft hair, a little paw towards us and two bright and shiny eyes, will always be able to bring back the good mood and warm even the hearts that have often cooled down.

Our day on the farm for this time is over, outside the sun is slowly setting towards the horizon and the animals are preparing to rest in their favorite huts.

In a corner of the barn there is a magnificent, thatched hut that the farmers have always used to watch over their animals, and for one night you too can experience the thrill of sleeping entirely immersed in the peace of nature.

Falling asleep on straw while breathing in the scent of hay is a highly soothing and relaxing experience.

There are no other noises except those of the horse and the donkey who together with you are looking for the best position to sleep, letting themselves go to the peace and quiet of the night.

Now it is time for everyone to close their eyes and let themselves go to sweet dreams.

If you like it, you can imagine having the tender cat you met before purring, or to caress the exceptionally soft hair of the puppy dog.

Let yourself go, there is no danger here.

The animals and nature will watch over you.

Do not think about anything.

Enjoy the smells of the countryside and the serenity that the animals have left imprinted inside you.

You can think of the moments you would like to relive the most, the moment you met the wagging puppy, or when you made the kitten purr, or when the horse started to trust you or when the donkey wanted to have a chat.

Breathe in the smell of straw and hay, enjoy the unique and special warmth that only a straw bed can give.

Connect with the universe and harmonize all the senses with nature and the creatures that populate it.

You have a special bed where you can relax and rest, soft and cozy like no other place in the world.

Here you can stay whenever you want, no one will wake you up or tell you that you overslept, there is no time or interruption of any kind.

You are tired and you want to think about nothing, but here you are in the ideal place to recover energy and get back active and positive.

Be at peace with the universe and you will see that the universe will also adapt to your desire for balance and stability. You will find the desired relief.

Stretch out like cats do, den like dogs do, and close your eyes.

Have a good rest.

Chapter 4 On the Soft Sand

Hi!

We are here together again to relax and take a moment all to ourselves.

Right now, all you must do is let go and stop accumulating your thoughts in a single tangled mess of negative knots and tangles.

Untie everything tightly on you, from your shoes to your belt to a necklace or in your hair, get comfortable and find a position where you don't have arms or legs that could hurt you.

If you want, you can put something warm on your belly or if you're getting ready for the night, slip under the covers and give the pillow the right shape so that with your head you can sink into something soft and comfortable.

I advise you to create a climate suitable for relaxation, maybe avoid keeping the lights on too loud, eliminate as much as you can the background noise, and make sure you have time for yourself, make sure that, as far as possible, no one comes to disturb you while you are focused on yourself and finding your inner serenity.

Before you start, take a deep breath, and let the air out along with the accumulated stress at the end of the day.

Do it one more time, inhale, and exhale.

Again, inhale and exhale, slowly.

Fill yourself with fresh air and positive vibrations.

Now that you have acclimatized yourself into a bubble of relaxation and relaxation, we're ready for another story that I hope will allow you to slip into sleep easily and with a smile on your face.

Are you ready?
Let's go!

On this occasion I want to take you to a beautiful and spectacular beach.

The most beautiful beach you have ever seen in the world, the one you have always imagined as the paradise on earth or the one where you would like to spend your annual vacation in peace and quiet or, why not, spend your retirement in a carefree and warm atmosphere.

Imagine you are already in the last hours of the afternoon, the sun is not bright, and the sky begins to turn pink, salmon and orange.

A walk on the beach can have numerous health benefits. Walking on the sand, in fact, promotes the cardiovascular system, improves blood flow, triggers endorphins, and reduces stress, giving a sense of tranquility and offering a relaxing effect.

When we walk barefoot on the sand, we give life to a natural massage that can reabsorb the blood that stagnates in the legs and feet. In this way the liquid is redistributed, the sense of tiredness and heaviness tends to disappear, and the aesthetic aspect also benefits.

In the foot but also in other parts of the body is reflected all over our body.

The plantar reflexology is traced back to ancient civilizations, especially oriental, but there is evidence that this technique was also practiced by pre-Columbian and Native American civilizations.

The natural stimulation of sand and stones, with their imperfections, is therefore a complete massage for the entire sole of the foot and therefore has a positive effect on all organs and glands.

Take off the shoes that bandage the foot and stay in contact with the bare earth gives a great feeling of freedom and well-being. This feeling of being supported, of being able to unload on the ground and the continuous massage under the feet improves our mood and calms the mind. A kind of self-therapy for body and mind.

It is relaxing, and we all have an inexhaustible need to relax, don't we?

Walking barefoot, wherever you are, on a safe and clean surface of course, allows the veins and muscles to relax, and it is a good habit both for children who find the stability they need to take their first steps, and for the elderly who keep their legs in training.

But now let's not focus too much attention on this practice that is good for the heart and mind, now let's go on imagining that we can walk barefoot on the most beautiful beach we have ever seen around sunset.

Beach walking reduces stress and has an almost meditative effect on our brain: it helps to free us from bad thoughts, brooding and emotions that do not allow us to feel good about ourselves.

Mental well-being is within reach of our feet when we are at the beach.

You are on the most iconic and majestic expanse of sand, one of the most beautiful beaches in the world. The colorful coral reef, located a short distance from the coast, keeps the ocean waves at bay, making it one of the most ideal places to dive into the warm waters of the ocean.

No matter what part of the Earth's hemisphere you are in, it is of no importance to determine the exact point on the map or precise geographical coordinates.

The only thing that is important to us now is that this beach is so big that it is as if you are the only tourist present, nobody sees you and judges you, you can wear a glossy magazine suit or - if you are in the right mood and it is in your style - walk completely naked.

White sand, clear water, an environment that makes you just want to stop and admire.

While you enjoy the softness of the sand and stretch your eyes to the horizon, following the slow and rhythmic movement of the waves, I will tell you some fantastic legends related to wonderful beaches in the world.

The first legend is set on a beach in southern Italy, a white and sunny beach, bathed by the Mediterranean Sea.

This is the romantic love story between Cristalda and Pizzomunno.

It is said that at the time when the current Italian town was just a village made up of scattered huts and inhabited by fishermen, there lived a tall and strong young man named Pizzomunno. In the same village also lived a young girl of rare beauty, with long sun colored hair named Cristalda. The two young men fell in love, loving each other madly without anything to separate them.

Both beautiful, shining for their strong and intense love that bound these two young people and loved to walk hand in hand along the beach.

Their love was so beautiful that it aroused the jealousies of the mermaids who inhabited the blue sea. They were jealous of that boy so beautiful and so devoted to his young love, they were jealous of that great love they had never experienced. Attracted by this, they tried in every way the young Pizzomunno, concurring and promising every kind of joy if only he would follow them. But he was sincerely in love with his Cristalda, refused any advances and remained faithful and united with his sweet beloved.

Blinded by such jealousy, they decided that they would no longer allow those two innocent boys to walk happily before their eyes. So it was that during a bright full moon evening, while the two young men were walking on the seashore and under the starry southern Italian sky, they kidnapped Cristalda and, with an evil spell, transformed Pizzomunno into stone.

There was not a day that the young Cristalda, transformed in turn into a mermaid, did not weep for her lost love. She cried so hard that the God of the sea, moved by compassion, allowed the two lovers to meet once every hundred years.

Since then, still today and forever, once every hundred years, those who live on the shores of that beautiful sea, can hear in the waves the cry of the two young people who meet again and for one day return to love each other.

Today you can admire the majesty of the Pizzomunno stacks on the homonymous Italian beach.

We stay in the Mediterranean to know some beaches and secrets of the island of Crete, Greece.

Shipwrecks and legends, ghosts and pirate adventures, bloody sieges and other tales set on five Greek beaches, including two Cretans. Not only turquoise waters and golden beaches; on these beaches disturbing stories cast their shadows on the sand, although most bathers, especially tourists, ignore them. In Greece, there are five beaches whose charm is enriched by their history and the anecdotes that are told about them.

Fragokastello, one of those five, is a beautiful beach in south-west Crete. This beach owes its charm and fame among tourists traveling to Crete to the shallow turquoise waters, but also to a curious legend.

A castle was built as protection from pirate attacks as well as the revolutionaries, and the stretch of sandy beach just below the castle saw the blood of countless battles spilled. In particular, one remembers the many Cretan fighters who were killed there during the revolution which saw the rebellious inhabitants of the region pitted against a Turkish army corps. Six hundred young Cretan boys heroically resisted the attack of eight thousand Turks for a week, but in the end many of them were killed, along with their leader. According to the legend, the bodies of the Greek warriors remained without burial until a strong wind carried the sand from the beach to cover their bodies pitifully.

Legend has it that from that date, on each anniversary of the battle, the ghosts of those killed in the massacre return to the beach for several nights and are visible at dawn. Between May and early June, anthropomorphic shadows, dressed in black and armed, on foot or on horseback, walk in line from the Church to the sea, where they disappear.

The ghosts of Frangokastello, which have never bothered anyone and do not frighten the locals or those who stay there on vacation, also have a name, Drosoulites, and the phenomenon has scientific explanations not fully verified that nothing detracts from the charm of the legend. The most reliable hypotheses to explain the apparitions are those of mirage and optical illusion.

The simplest explanation could be that of the optical illusion caused by the evaporation of dew in the morning. The haze generated by this evaporation, a phenomenon particularly perceptible at the end of May, would take the form of several figures that the imagination would come to interpret as human features.

According to another explanation, no less fascinating than ghost theory, this phenomenon is due to a mirror image of the northern coast of Africa. The figures of the Drosulites would be the shadows of the desert camel drivers!

Although they are authoritative sources talking about the phenomenon and many people claim to have witnessed the appearance of the Drosulites on the beach, there is no photographic or video document that proves its existence.

Another story is that of Elafonisi, one of the most beautiful and famous beaches in all of Greece; its name, written sometimes with different spelling, creates a misunderstanding for those who know little about the language and history of Crete, diverting the mind from the true origin of the name and its true history.

The beach is characterized by an exotic aspect, separated from the rest of Crete by a thin strip of shallow sea where you can walk, currently has a name that brings to mind a word that in Greek means "deer"... but the island, which is certainly not and has never been populated by deer, should actually be called in another way and with a similar word meaning "spoils", because the pirates hid their "spoils" right here.

If the fact that it was an island of pirates was not enough to increase its charm, we must remember that on Elafonisi was written a high black page of the history of Crete: on Easter Sunday of the one thousand eight hundred and twenty-four the Turks slaughtered in an ambush about eight hundred people including women, elders and soldiers, as reprisal for their rebellion against the Ottoman domination. The blood of the killed dyed the pearly sand of the island red, the survivors were sold as slaves in the markets of the East.

Another historical detail on the island of Elafonisi, also quite macabre, is the shipwreck in front of the island of an Austrian steamship, the Imperatrix, which occurred due to a storm in the night between the twenty-first and twenty-two of February of the nineteenth century. The wreck of the sunken ship is still on the bottom of the sea, stranded between the cliffs in front of the island at a shallow depth. In a position accessible by boat on days of calm sea, it offers suggestive images to scuba diving enthusiasts.

But do you know that there is even a beach of stars?

Don't you believe it?

Well, it is the truth.

In Japan you can walk, literally, among the stars!

To live this unusual experience, you just must leave and visit at least one of the Japanese islands where there are Hoshizuna no Hama, or "beaches with sand of stars". You can also do it, as we have become accustomed to, by being comfortably relaxed in an armchair or cuddled under the covers in your comfortable bed.

Imagine seeing that in the Hatoma, Iriomote and Taketomi islands, all belonging to Okinawa prefecture, the southernmost prefecture of Japan, there are beaches whose sand also contains grains in the form of microscopic white stars.

What are stars made of? You may be wondering.

The star-shaped sand grains of Japanese beaches resemble incredible miniature works of art but have not been sculpted by an artist.

They are the shells of some microscopic foraminiferous protozoa, the Baculogypsina sphaerulata, which have between five and six pointed arms that help them move from one place to another and anchor themselves to the algae through which they feed.

These tiny stars are among the oldest fossils that man can find and touch, in fact a large number of scientists believe that there are traces of their existence dating back five hundred million years ago and for this reason they are also analyzing them to study the climate change that has suffered the planet Earth during the various geological eras.

The shape of these exoskeletons made of calcium carbonate, makes these shells no larger than a millimeter. A curious marine heritage that the force of the waves of the ocean and the wind bring to shore on the beaches.

The moment when it is easier to find so many starry grains by the sea?

Obviously after tides and typhoons that exponentially increase the concentration of these tiny star-shaped shells.

Millions of tourists from all over the world come to these Japanese islands in search of the Star Sand Beaches.

Some souvenir stores sometimes give a small bag of it as a gift to those who store locally. The local community is so proud of this phenomenon that to avoid that some tourists do not know that, mixed with the classic grains of white sand, there are billions of "small stars" there are even signs with a big yellow star in the center that remind us to look for the "stars" on the seashore, where it is easier to find them.

There is a fascinating legend that has belonged to the Japanese folk tradition for many centuries that explains the "heavenly" origin of these small stars.

The sand of stars would be born from the meeting between the Polar Star and the Southern Cross, stars that are at the antipodes of the firmament.

Tradition says that the small stars would be the offspring of the two stars and would have been generated right in the sea off Okinawa but that a ferocious sea snake would have immediately killed them, abandoning their small skeletons in the waters of the Ocean.

After walking along the shoreline of our imaginary beach of fine white sand, soft and wet by warm, calm and crystal-clear waters, you can see a beautiful hammock just between two trunks of palm trees lying on the sand and of course you are invited to try it.

A small curiosity: the hammock was a sort of suspended bed used by pre-Columbian people, made of a cloth supported by intertwined ropes, whose ends hung from two trees or inside the huts. In this way it escaped from the sultry heat thanks to a better ventilation of the body.

The great explorers such as Christopher Columbus and Amerigo Vespucci, knew it during the one thousand five hundred and, in addition to bringing it to Europe, used it on ships for the rest of sailors.

The origin of the hammock therefore, that is its invention, goes up again to a period of almost a millennium ago among the inhabitants of South America.

The high temperature of the place, therefore the need to be able to sleep or take a siesta in a shady place, or outdoors at night, probably were the motivational levers that generated such an ingenious invention.

In fact, the possibility to fix it between two trees goes to conjugate both the advantages, that means shade and being outdoors in an airy place.

The notions that have come down to us tell us that the original material for them artisan production of the hammock was the bark of the trees, later the Sisal (Agave sisalana) because it is a material that has resistant characteristics of elasticity and flexibility, and then get to the fabric of cotton and therefore to the various possibilities of coloring.

Since the discovery of America, thanks to Christopher Columbus, the hammock has come down to in Europe and thanks to the ease of fixing and use has become a bed of rest also on ships. In some cases, has been exploited even in the galleys of the United Kingdom.

For travelers of yesteryear, accustomed to having to sleep at the bedside proved to be an indispensable baggage, also for the fact that allows you to easily stay relieved from the ground to the desired height, away from insects, moisture, from any puddles of water.

Thanks to the ease of transport, fixing and use, the relative inexpensiveness of the product, the fame and use of the hammock have spread all over the world.

We have not yet talked about one of the most famous features of the hammock: the rocking! Snuggling on a hammock is particularly restful, thanks to the rocking, which according to some would bring back to the neonatal dimension of the cradle.

Some scholars have published research that states that the hammock reconciles deep sleep, while according to other scientists the research is not exhaustive. On one fact, however, everyone agrees: swinging, you fall asleep first. Which is the right rhythm to facilitate the transition from waking to sleep? An oscillation every four seconds, therefore absolute slowness.

After all, the light rocking promotes relaxation, and stimulates some regenerating naps.

I would say it is just right for us.

Well, now we sit in the hammock, which is cozy and immediately embraces us in its comfort.

Around us there are no sounds other than the relaxing sounds of a paradisiacal beach. We hear the relaxing sound of the waves breaking on the shoreline at a slow and regular rhythm. There is something extremely reassuring in this repetitive and constant sound, it is an element that stays still and never tires of being heard.

The sound of the lapping of the waves contains in itself all the frequencies audible to the human ear and for this reason it is called "white noise".

You see, the noise of the sea has minimal and gradual volume variations that do not trigger a state of vigilance necessary to defend against possible dangers.

The rhythm of brain activity slows down, while you let yourself go completely.

The noise that the wind makes between the leaves of the palm trees seems to have no meaning,

and yet, if you listen carefully, you hear in that rustle the invitation of the wind to let yourself be rocked.

The wind begins to swing your hammock in a gentle, slow, relaxing way.

Your hammock is supported by two palm trees that will watch over you like two strong warriors.

We have often seen images of hurricanes that show us all kinds of destruction: houses collapsed, floods, trees torn apart... many, but not the palm trees, which for the most part can withstand the fury of the wind and remain standing. Have you ever wondered how these plants can withstand even the strongest hurricanes?

Palms have many roots: they are relatively short, but they develop radially in the soil and can anchor very strongly to the ground.

The trunk of the palm trees also consists of many small bundles of woody material, which can be imagined as an electric cable consisting of many wires.

Unlike other plants, such as oak for example, palms are not able to support huge weights, such as large branches and thick foliage, but on the other hand they have considerable flexibility.

Most trees have a thick foliage of branches and twigs and a large number of leaves to capture as much light as possible from the sun, but this produces a remarkable sail effect when they are hit by strong winds, which can pull the plant uprooted. Palm trees, on the other hand, have exceptionally large leaves with a flexible central "spine": they look like huge feathers. When the weather is good, the foliage produces a thick foliage, but in strong winds the leaves fold in the direction of the wind: in this way they offer less resistance and can more easily withstand even the strongest hurricanes.

As you can see, you are completely safe.

Now let yourself go to the rocking hammock slightly moved by the wind. A light, warm, soft, and caressing wind.

Let yourself listen to the sound of the sea breaking on the shore, interrupted only by the singing of some seagull.

Do you like seagulls? I like these sea birds very much.

Do you want to know what is told about the origin of seagulls?

There is an ancient agricultural legend that seagulls are the souls of sailors who died at sea and those who kill or drive them away attract the wrath of the Lord.

In Acropolis in the eighteenth century there was a famine and a serious pestilence.

The only food not infected was fish. The fishermen, however, if, intent on fishing, crossed unknown boats, suddenly returned to the port, to avoid any form of contagion.

Then there was the stormy sea for several days, which prevented the fishermen to set sail and dedicate themselves to fishing, necessary for the sustenance of the population in that period of food shortage. Later, despite the persistence of bad weather conditions, which made it dangerous to venture on fishing trips, the fishermen, faced with the dramatic conditions of their families who were on the verge of starvation, decided to undertake the same fishing trip. The youngest and strongest ones set sail with three boats, keeping a distance between the three boats such that they could communicate with each other.

They cast their nets, hoping for abundant fishing. Their destiny, however, was now marked: a tremendous wave swept the boats, throwing them into the depths of the sea. On the beach adjacent to the port, the women waited in vain for their heroic men. St. Peter and St. Paul witnessed the dramatic event. Feeling pity for the unfortunate sailors, they transformed them into seagulls, birds with beautiful white wings, storm warnings to the fishermen who go out to sea.

The seagulls that fly over the port of Acropolis are the souls of the dead fishermen and with their flights they indicate the arrival of a goodbye or a storm. They are docile and tame birds, to which the fishermen often offer food as a sign of affection and familiarity.

Perhaps even those you hear singing are gentle souls of ancient and brave sailors. Do not be frightened, they too are here to protect your sleep and watch over you.

You are in a beautiful place, without clock, without phone, without agenda, without timetables. You are here because you deserve it.

Everyone knows that you need it, and they want you to rest and relax, nothing else.

A last glance is dedicated to the romantic sunset that is painting around.

The sky is tinged with lilac, salmon, orange, and pink. The ocean has become impenetrable, so dark that it seems almost black. The waves, with their golden reflections, began to dance softly. And the sun, little by little, came down with an imperceptible movement, and with each step things were colored with different and new colors.

The sunset, if you think about it, in art and literature often appears as a metaphor, the light that disappears and the shadow that invades the entire visual field sometimes transmit melancholy and sadness, a feeling of loneliness and abandonment, sometimes even anxiety and fear. But, thinking about it, in reality the moment of sunset is not sad at all: its splendid colors always manage to enchant the senses and the mind, the play of shadows and light seem to open the door to an unknown and fantastic world.

Sometimes, the image of the sunset evokes in us a feeling of nostalgia and regret, as inexorable symbol of the passing time, but we must stop bonding to what tends to the negative and leave room for beauty, yes, looking only at its beauty we will always be able to overcome any negative feeling, opening the way to creativity and imagination.

Around you, very quietly and slowly, silence descends just as the sun does, which will soon disappear behind the clouds just above the horizon.

Look for an ideal position so as not to miss this special moment, that of colors and transform the magic of the instant into an emotion.

The sea, unlike the sky, gradually takes on colder colors with colder tones.

The colors and the light are in continuous attenuation, soon they will give way to the evening.

A distant ship on the horizon turns on the lights on board and prepares for the night.

Gradually the sea stretches out, as if it gave up exhausted at nightfall.

You can still feel the wind blowing on your face, lukewarm from the west.

And there you are, rocking quietly and relaxed in your private hammock, enchanted by the beauty of the sky. Feel your cheeks barely red from the sun taken during the walk on the soft sand.

It could be one of those special moments to take inside, even on winter days that all look the same, under the warm comforter and inside a cup of steaming tea.

Breathe in the rhythm of the sea.

Inhale the typical smell of salt and maybe some exotic sunscreen that someone forgot near your hammock.

Keep rocking, completely abandoned.

Just enjoy the sensation of the sunset that changes gradually towards the evening, preparing the stage for the protagonist of the night: the moon, with its company of galaxies and stars.

This night imagine you are right on that beach. Your personal and perfect beach. You are on your soft, enveloping, and welcoming hammock, placed between two solid palm trees.

You do not feel any cold or humidity, you feel great, in tune with the wild and paradisiacal beach.

Breathe and relax, let yourself go rocking.

The ropes that support the hammock also produce a slight rhythmic squeaking, which accompanies and reconciles sleep together with the waves that break on the shore.

Relax and enjoy the lightheartedness that the Caribbean setting offers you.

Your beach will always be there, unchanged, and ready to give you perfect isolation. You are in a safe and quiet place.

Every end of the day the sun will merge with the horizon of the sea giving shows of an extraordinary beauty, every evening with similar colors and yet never identical to the previous ones.

The clouds will take away any negative thoughts, letting themselves be swept away by the wind.

Rocking in a hammock makes you feel good. You can swing as long as you want, this place is all yours and you can stay and listen and rest to the soothing sounds offered by the beach.

Little by little a golden, white, and magnificent moon rises high in the sky.

Its reflection makes the waves silvery and recalls ancient legends of sea gods and mermaids in love.

You can fall asleep peacefully, lulled by the warm wind and watched over by the palm trees.

Your sleep will be deep and regenerating.

You can dream of Caribbean beaches, fine white sand and warm, crystal clear waters.

Close your eyes and imagine enjoying the warmth that emanates from the sand still warm for the sun.

Let yourself go.

Breathe and imagine yourself in this enchanting and heavenly place.

It is okay, you are okay, and you can take your mind off it and let yourself slip into a sweet sleep full of dreams and Caribbean places.

Swing, let yourself swing.

Let the rocking rock your sleep like the sleep of a newborn baby while being cradled in its innocent cradle.

Sleep and keep rocking, do not worry about anything.

Everything is great.

Sleep now, let yourself swing and sleep.

Enjoy your sleep.

Chapter 5 Herb Is A Magic Rug

Hello, welcome.

We are here to slip together into a new world of fantasy and relaxation, thanks to stories where everything is possible and where you feel infinitely calm, serene, protected.

In these pages I will try to create for you a perfect atmosphere where you can heal your heart from the wounds you may be carrying inside, or to have some relief.

Between these lines there is no anxiety, no stress or worry.

In here you feel good, you become one with the comfortable and warm mattress of your bed, or with the sofa where you snuggled up with a soft blanket, or with the armchair that envelops you and supports your head during reading.

As I hope I have got used to doing by now, let yourself go first.

Breathe deeply and try to prevent anxiety and worries from slipping into your sleep conciliation moment.

Make sure like other times that you can have this moment all to yourself, that possibly no one comes to disturb you or interrupt your relaxation and total relaxation.

Make yourself comfortable, adjust the lights so that they are warm and enveloping, maybe light an abatjour or a candle, but make sure not to leave it lit if you fall asleep before the end of this story, you can also use a candle with relaxing scents.

Make sure that you are neither hungry nor thirsty, and above all not to be in a hurry, that you have done your needs in the bathroom and that you no longer need to leave your position until you are completely relaxed and fall asleep like a baby.

In the other stories we walked in a beautiful park in the fall season, and we walked on a fabulous Caribbean beach, on this occasion I would like to take you by the hand and let you discover something you probably did when you were a cheerful and carefree child: walking on the grass barefoot.

Of course, at this moment you will do it simply by being comfortable in your favorite place and following my words. Using the power of imagination and letting yourself go completely, waiting maybe to actually do it tomorrow.

This kind of contact with the Earth is an increasingly rare experience today but know that when you are very tired and need to draw new energy, you can look for a meadow near where you are, turn off the phone and take a nice barefoot walk for at least a quarter of an hour!

Wherever you are, however, walking barefoot gives you a feeling of widespread well-being. Do you know why?

Already Abbot Kneipp, one of the historical fathers of Naturopathy, advised as a panacea to walk barefoot early in the morning on the grass wet with dew. This custom may perhaps seem anachronistic for us, who live locked up in the city, tight in the gray walls and asphalt, but in reality, we have forgotten that the earth has always been "mother" and source of a regenerative force, capable of recharging and reharmonizing ourselves, especially when we are overworked by an excess of intellectual work, when our batteries are exhausted, or we feel overloaded with stress.

It seems that the earth emits an energy current that represents a natural regeneration system.

During evolution man has walked barefoot and slept on the ground, thus receiving all the benefits of the sweet electricity of the soil.

The modern way of life has separated man from this omnipresent flow of subtle energy.

We wear shoes with insulating rubber that block the flow and, of course, we no longer sleep on the ground as we used to.

However, research is now showing that "grounding" brings many health benefits: it increases vitality, harmonizes, and stabilizes the body's basic biological rhythms, reduces chronic inflammation and pain, and promotes better sleep.

We can get an immediate recharging of energy simply by walking barefoot on a lawn.

When you walk barefoot you absorb millions of electrons that intercept free radicals. In this way the body can detoxify and as a result the blood becomes more fluid.

Moreover, it is not just a feeling of well-being. Some time ago, a well-known brand of shoes made a thorough investigation into a South American tribe that still lived off hunting by running and walking barefoot. The tribe was known because its members were able to run amazingly fast and for a very long time. This is because running barefoot is better.

Imagine now walking in a forest or in an open field, in the coolness of the branches of the trees, with the pleasant air of spring that warms your skin, awakened after the rigidity of winter. Even plants are reborn from the torpor of the cold and nature rediscovers its vocation as a generator of life: we feel at one with "Mother Nature" all around us. At this point, what could be better to try?

Well, now imagine that you can do it barefoot, free, in direct contact with the earth, with water, no obstacles between you and the dewy soil, the soft grass. A grass that becomes like a magic carpet.

Man needs direct contact with nature.

Going barefoot puts us in a sort of new state of mind that is usually reserved only for a few special moments of relaxation...this is what happens when you start going barefoot. Then imagine you are on a green and tender turf, and it will be a real treat.

The exercises to strengthen the body and relax the mind (yoga, tai chi, martial arts) are also typically done barefoot.

Even our feet express with an unpleasant smell simply their discomfort to be closed in the shoes!

Continuing our pleasant walk, we meet some flowers and plants that you might be interested in getting to know better.

Let us imagine that it is spring, the season in which nature triumphs.

We first meet a lavender stain. Lavandula is a plant native to the Mediterranean countries and is particularly suitable for forming low hedges or avenues borders.

It has leaves typical of the species only narrower and more intense green.

The flowers are carried by long blue spikes, very perfumed, which open in summer.

There are many varieties of this species on the market with flowers of various colors from red to white to blue.

Together with other aromatic and medicinal plants such as Valerian, it is very appreciated for its relaxing effects on the nervous system. The essential oil is in fact particularly effective in reducing stress, insomnia, and palpitations. Its valuable but delicate scent relaxes the nerves and naturally promotes a state of general well-being and relaxation.

Now imagine that you can sink your nostrils into a beautiful lavender bush and smell its relaxing scent.

Do you like lavender? I will tell you some interesting things about it.

The scent of lavender attracts the bees, which produce an excellent aromatic honey, while mosquitoes don't like it, so it is advisable to rub lavender water on sultry summer evenings to cool down and at the same time avoid annoying stings.

In ancient times lavender was used not only for its perfume and personal hygiene but also as a disinfectant: in the Middle Ages and until the eighteenth century, lavender was sprinkled and rubbed floors using it as a disinfectant and was used for the preparation of potpourri to perfume the house.

The etymological derivation of the name leaves no doubt and recalls the use that the Romans made of this plant: they used it to perfume bath water and as a detergent.

The ear is also considered an amulet against misfortunes and demons and is also said to be a talisman to bring prosperity and fertility.

Lavender is the astral essence of the zodiac sign of Aries.

In the language of flowers, Lavender can have two distinct and contradictory meanings.

The first meaning refers to an ancient tradition that tells that lavender was used in ancient times against snake bites and recommended to find it on wounds after letting it macerate in water. It was therefore considered an antidote, but it was also said that inside its bush's snakes nested there, especially asps, so the ancient people approached them with great caution. From this belief derived its meaning in the language of flowers that is to say "distrust".

The second meaning of lavender is linked to milder feelings and giving lavender as a gift would mean "your memory is my only happiness".

By now you know that I like to tie the elements I tell you about to stories and legends, to make you fly with fantasy. Well, there is a beautiful legend also linked to lavender.

In Provence, in the south of France, there are many legends related to lavender. In the area Valensole, in particular, they tell the story of Lavandula, a fairy with blond hair and blue eyes born in the wild mountain of Lure. It is said that the fairy took a book of landscapes to choose the place to live. In front of the page that showed the valleys of Provence all arid and without nature, she started to cry. Lavandula's tears, falling on the book, stained it with blue hues, to cover the damage he had done, the fairy took a piece of sky and spread it over Provence.

Since then, according to legend, Provence is covered with lavender and all the girls have blue eyes like those of Lavandula.

There are other legends related to lavender and one of the oldest is that of Venus and its magical rites of love, it is said that the Goddess used this plant so that its scent attracted men, ensuring not only love, but also happiness, protection, purification and joy. From here the tradition wants that some ears of lavender are placed inside the trousseau of the future bride to wish her happiness and prosperity.

Right next to this lilac-colored stain of lavender bushes individuals of the other wonderful flowers and the same color, are the lilac flowers.

The lilac color is considered a light and bright purple that can reach almost white. Its meaning is the awakening of the soul and represents the control of rationality over emotionality. It is the conjunction of body and mind.

It is much loved by the female world and by brides. It is often associated with homosexuality because it is obtained by mixing blue, the male color, with red, pink, the female color. In general, it is a symbol of eroticism and pleasure.

The origins of color date back to ancient times. A legend says that the fairy people lived among the lilac flowers. Other tales report that the flowers were used to protect people from darkness and temptation. In Greek mythology it is said that the god Hephaestus crowned himself with lilac flowers to seduce Aphrodite.

Along with pink, it is a spring color because lilac flowers are among the first to bloom in this season. If you think, for example, of lavender or wisteria flowers around a pergola, you will immediately feel a sensation of freshness and rebirth, typical emotions of this season.

Another ancient Greek legend about lilac flowers tells that the young Pan, the god of woods and fields, one fine morning met the beautiful nymph Syringe. Fascinated by her grace and beauty, he wanted to talk to her. But she was afraid and ran away. Pan tried to reach her, but he met a fragrant lilac bush, which had blocked his way ... Pan started crying that he had lost the nymph and from then on, he began to wander through the forests and do charity work, and the name of Syringe became the Latin name for lilac.

Another legend tells that lilacs appeared when spring had made the snow disappear from the field and raised the sun in the sky. The sun then met the rainbow and together they had crossed the sky. The spring had collected some sun rays and mixed them with the colors of the rainbow and then started to put them on the ground. When spring came to the north, she was left with only two colors left, white and purple, colors that indicated the spring of the Scandinavian countries. Then the spring threw the colors of lilacs on a flowery bush, remaining only the white color and scattered them on the ground. In the places where the white color fell on the bushes, white lilacs grew. Lilac takes its name from the Greek word "Syrinx" which means flute since the shepherds built the small flute from the lilac tree. In Russia, on the other hand, it was also called "Sinel", which derives from the word blue because blue was the main color of the plant.

I hope these legends about flowers are making you smile pleasantly, they are a way like any other to allow us to find the right connection with nature and with elements that now, living in cities, we find in our hands more and more rarely.

You walk a little bit more in the fresh and soft grass, which softens your steps and cuddles your feet, until a wonderful flower called white lily comes out.

As always, I have a little legend in store for you.

It is said that the white lily was born from a drop of milk that fell to the ground during Hera's breast-feeding to Hercules. In fact, since Hercules was the son of the god Zeus and the mortal Alcmene, Zeus demanded that Hercules was nursed from the breast of his wife, the goddess Hera, to become immortal. While she was sleeping, they put the baby on her chest and when she nursed him, some drops of milk ended up in the universe creating the Milky Way, and the drops that fell to earth were called white lily.

According to the Bible, the Easter lily grew in the Garden of Gethsemane, where Judas had betrayed Jesus. According to the legend, the white lily grew in the spot where Jesus' tears and sweat fell in the last moments of his life. The white lily is the symbol of purity of the Blessed Virgin Mary.

Another legend has it that when the tomb of the Virgin Mary was visited three days after her funeral, a whole bunch of magnificent white lilies appeared.

In a different female context, the lily had an important place in Adam and Eve's Paradise. According to legend, when Eve left the Garden of Eden, she shed tears of repentance and from those tears of repentance the lilies sprang.

The lilies, finally, were the signs of protection of the Knights Templar.

Sometimes next to the lilies we find equally tall and beautiful companions, flowers that stand out among others for their tall, proud, and elegant posture. I am talking about irises.

Can a little curiosity about irises be lacking?

The iris is a plant rich in history and symbolism because it has always been appreciated in all civilizations. Frescoes depicting irises were found at the walls of the temple of Amon at Karnak (ancient Thebes) in Egypt, and in the botanical garden of Pharaoh

Tuthmosis III. It is said that the first species of irises were transported to Egypt by Pharaoh from Syria.

The ancient Greeks identified the iris with Iris, the messenger of the Gods, handmaid of Hera, who was the vessel that allowed men to receive the messages of the Gods. According to mythology Iris to descend among men slipped on the rainbow (hence the genesis of the name).

The iris was the coat of arms of Clovis the First, king of the Salian Franks, the second historically established ruler of the Merovingian dynasty, who had it depicted on flags, shields, armor and tapestries, after receiving this flower in a dream from an angel, who had appeared to honor the event of his conversion to Christianity, which occurred after the victory of the Battle of Tolbiac in which the sovereign and his army drove the Alemanni from the upper Rhine, in the year four hundred and ninety-six.

It is known that the coat of arms of the city of Florence, in Italy, and of Louis the Seventh is a lily but in reality, originally in both cases it had to be an iris. According to many historical data, in fact, Louis the Seventh had decided to include an iris in his royal coat of arms, but for this reason the flower was called fleur de Louis (Louis flower), unfortunately its pronunciation is very similar to fleur de lys which means lily and probably for this reason over the years the two names were confused and the coat of arms of Louis the Seventh became the lily. The same fate happened to the coat of arms of the city of Florence.

In the one thousand nineteen hundred and fifty-four in Florence was created the Garden of the Iris, in Piazzale Michelangelo born with the aim of giving hospitality to the annual international competition for the best varieties of irises.

In the artistic sphere, many times the white iris has taken the place of the lily in paintings dedicated to the Madonna.

In the language of flowers and plants, the iris generally symbolizes good news, although its meaning may change depending on the variety.

After admiring the magnificent white lilies and splendid irises, can we fail to imagine a magnificent rose garden?

You can imagine the varieties that most appeal to you: red, white, yellow, pink, or even blue. All of them of a fairy beauty and fragrant one of the most beloved perfumes in the world.

The rose is the flower to give par excellence and each variety carries a different message. The rose has been a symbol of love, devotion, admiration, beauty, and perfection for centuries. The rose also symbolizes the secret and reveals it with delicacy.

The well closed rosebud of the Rose also embodies female chastity while the blossoming Rose represents youthful beauty.

In Roman mythology, the Lovers' Rose was the flower sacred to Venus and has remained to this day as an expression of deep and passionate love.

In the Greek and Roman world instead, the rose was associated with the myth of Adonis and Aphrodite: the goddess, in love with the young hunter, there is nothing she can do to save him from death caused by the attack of a wild boar. In rescuing her beloved, Aphrodite wounds herself with brambles and her blood makes red roses bloom. Zeus, moved by the pain of the goddess, allows Adonis to live four months in Hades, four in the world of the living, and four more where he would have preferred: for this reason, the rose is considered a symbol of love that overcomes death and also of rebirth.

In the language of flowers, the dog rose symbolizes both poetry and independence. It is even mentioned in the Bible: Judas probably used the dog rose tree to commit suicide; again, Jesus' crown of thorns was presumably made from the branches of this shrub.

The Romans celebrated the Rosalia, linked to the cult of the dead, in a period between the eleventh of May and the fifteenth of July: this feast of roses was transmitted to the Christian world, where Pentecost is also called "Easter of roses". The rose was also present in the cult of Dionysus, for the belief that it prevented drunks from revealing their secrets.   In the iconography of Christian mysticism, the rose, for its beauty, its perfume, for the mystery of its shape appreciated since time immemorial and for its color mostly red, the very ancient symbol of love, indicates the cup that collected the blood of Christ or the transformation of the drops of this blood or the wounds of Christ himself.

Also, do not forget, the scent of roses has always fascinated us. Homer had Aphrodite anoint Hector's corpse with essential rose oil, while Dicrurids and Pliny already described the preparation. In the annals of Emperor Akbar, however, written in the sixteenth century, the discovery of the essential oil of roses was attributed to the wife of Emperor Jahangir, who had the essence that floated in the canals of the imperial gardens, fed with rose water, then called it the scent of Jahangir in honor of her husband.

But the rose is not the only flower symbol of love, there is also the tulip.

The tulip is in fact one of the flowers that most of all symbolizes love, so much so that its birth is linked to an ancient Persian legend that tells of a sentimental disappointment.

The name tulip comes from the Turkish 'tullband' which means turban, probably because of its characteristic shape. It is a flower very present in Turkish culture and in many fairy tales, among the most famous 'The Thousand and One Nights'.

During the reign of Sultan Suleiman, the Magnificent, the tulip reached its maximum popularity, so much so that from his court were exported to Vienna, then to Holland and England.

The red tulip is associated with love, and according to some tales, the sultan dropped one of these flowers at the feet of one of the women of the harem to indicate the chosen one.

Another ancient Persian tradition tells of the origin of tulips:

Once upon a time there was a young man named Shirin in love with the beautiful Ferhad, a love reciprocated but destined to be broken.

According to legend Shirin had left in search of fortune, leaving his beloved alone and waiting for him.

For a long time, the woman had waited for his return, but unfortunately one day while wandering in search of the boy, she fell on sharp stones and cried with the knowledge that she would die without seeing Shirin again.

Her tears mixed with the blood and falling drop after drop on the ground, they turned into beautiful red flowers: tulips.

Since then, all the springs of these flowers have bloomed again in memory of this unhappy love.

Giving a red tulip is like saying "I love you and I will love you forever", the violet tulip indicates modesty, a statement yes, but not too demanding.

The yellow tulip is, instead, suitable for a sunny and carefree love.

I hope you had fun learning about many legends that revolve around the world of flowers. Maybe some are better known than others, but all of them are certainly curious and full of exciting and strong characters.

The secret of all these characters is that they have completely let go of their emotions, they have lived their feelings to the point of being overwhelmed by them.

So even now I ask you to let yourself go to the emotions that these stories instill in you, occupying your mind with images of ancient worlds, of colorful and wonderful flowers, of pure and simple beauty.

Our barefoot walk is almost coming to an end, the blue spring sky dotted with nice little clouds is preparing the scene for the moon and its dancers, the stars.

Imagine you can lie down freely in the grass. In your imagination you do not feel any coolness, only the soft embrace of the turf that supports you better than any mattress.

Maybe you cross your legs and join your hands as a pillow under your head and look above you.

Climbing this tree is the last beautiful flower of which I want to tell you the legend.

I am talking about "Morning glory", or bells, beautiful flowers from Central America and Mexico. It is a semi rustic species and is characterized by heart-shaped leaves and blue flowers tending to purple in the shape of a trumpet with the central part shaded white. These cute flowers open in the morning and turn their beautiful blue flower towards the sun, make them reborn and decorate whatever you plant near them. The mysterious fact of morning glory is that they close their flower in the late afternoon and apparently go to sleep until the next morning.

According to a legend, a beautiful princess loved to sit among the flowers in her garden. But she was very delicate of health and so she had to return to the palace before the day got too hot.

In this way she could not admire some of the varieties of flowers in the garden because they opened only when the sun was shining on them. This made the princess incredibly sad, because it is known that princesses have a noble heart. One day when she returned to the palace, she started crying. As she walked her tears fell on the floor and every tear that touched the ground turned into a small seed. A few weeks later, when the princess was walking in her garden, one morning early in the morning, she was very surprised when she suddenly noticed a beautiful new flower that had been born and was growing and was inhaling on the spiral-shaped garden wall with its beautiful branches and leaves all around the trees and arches. Her heart filled with joy and the name "The Beauty of the Morning" was given to the flower on the one hand because it had emerged from the tears from the beautiful blue eyes of the princess, and on the other because it had given her so much joy in her morning walks.

Wouldn't you like to wake up fresh and full of energy early tomorrow morning to see these magnificent open flowers?

To do that, though, we need to rest now.

You are in a lovely place, surrounded by fragrant lavender, charming lilacs, seductive roses, and beautiful tulips, and the "morning glory" will watch over you while you sleep together.

You can also imagine that you are in turn a blue bell. You can feel on yourself the sensation of the petals closing to protect your inner heart through the blanket that shelters you over your shoulders or the curtains that close the windows of your house.

And tomorrow morning you will greet the sun.

It will be a serene and graceful rest from the moon, you will not feel cold and you will not have any worries, because the petals protect you and the grass is soft and welcomes you as it welcomes its fruits, trees and flowers.

Tomorrow morning you can wake up to the sound of a melodic concert of birds, with the faint light of the morning making its way through the cracks in the branches of a centuries-old tree and you will finally feel relieved, at peace with yourself and the world.

Imagine the feeling of well-being felt as you close your eyes after a long day of appointments, losing your gaze on a sky of blue flowers, and wake up discovering that you are still surrounded by so much beauty.

Many scholars of nature say that the best time to walk through nature is in the early hours of the day because only then can you capture the scents, colors and freshness of nature, perhaps in a drop of dew laid on a small bud that stubbornly struggles to see the sunlight.

I have to say that they are right, even if in the cool spring days wandering around a park is as regenerating as looking for a secular tree in autumn or new blooms in summer, expelling nature at dawn or dusk gives different emotions depending on how the sunlight moves.

However, many of us could be intimidated by the idea of spending a whole night outdoors, so our rest under the "morning glory" and among the flowers could simply turn into a nap.

Often you yawn after walking and accumulate tiredness, therefore, leave your imaginary self or yourself about to fall asleep before the night or maybe at another time of the day when you felt the need is that you can finally let yourself go should be easier.

Breathe and let yourself be enveloped by the blue petals of the flower bells that fall asleep.

Let your body relax as much as possible, allowing your eyes to gently close and let your mind gracefully slide into the garden of dreams.

Your breath welcomes the fresh scent of the earth and freshly cut grass, the ancestral scent of the pure and living earth.

You can feel safe and protected by nature.

This grass is clean, dry, and safe.

Nature is happy to be able to embrace you on its land, it just wants you to relax and fall asleep in peace with it.

Everything is calm, velvety, silent.

Weed gives you relief.

You feel protected and well-liked, warm, ready to dream.

Nothing but the sun at dawn will wake you up, but only if you want it, because otherwise the majestic trees will create a roof of branches with their fronds and allow you to sleep until you feel full of positive energy.

You feel that you are finally freeing yourself from all the pressures that create anxiety and disturbances.

Touching the earth is a physical but also a mental action. It is an act of reunification and surrender, of seeking balance.

We touch the earth to let go of the idea of being disconnected from everything else, and to remind ourselves that we are the Earth and part of Life.

When we touch the Earth, we become small, with the humility and simplicity of a child.

And like a child, without worries and with the sweet and innocent breath of a newborn mixed with the purity of nature, he now slips into a deep and enveloping sleep.

If as a child you have never tried to sleep outdoors or in a campsite, this is the right opportunity to try and enjoy those wonderful sensations.

Let yourself go into the universe, let yourself be embraced by Mother Nature.

Sleep peacefully now, dream and rest in harmony with heaven and earth.

Chapter 6 Let's Sweeten Our Lives

If we should think about one of the happy and carefree moments of our childhood, we will certainly find among them a memory involving something sweet, maybe a birthday cake, a wake-up call with maple syrup pancakes, or a hot chocolate during a winter afternoon, a cream cupcake as a reward after a particularly hard day, or a homemade tart baked with mom or grandma.

We can also pause for a moment, here and now, to dig up that happy memory if we have one that we remember easily and perhaps frequently enough, or, if we don't, we can imagine it as always.

I am telling you about these sweet memories because in this story I would like you to relive the serene and peaceful feelings that hover around them. For a moment, I would like you to return to that happy child, to find within you that innocent enthusiasm and pure joy felt after blowing the candles on your birthday cake or after licking the chocolate off your lips.

I realize that thinking about food might be a bad idea before we fall asleep, in general it is always better not to go to bed or lie down just after eating a big meal, and even worse is to try to rest distracted by hunger bites.

In this case, however, I would like you not to think so much of sweets as a time to binge or to unleash your gluttony, but rather in relation to the moments of happiness and joy, of lightness and festivity that bind to sugary food.

This is not the place to discuss diets or what is good or bad, how harmful to the teeth and various eating disorders, I am talking about sweetness in the purest and most authentic state of the term.

I even advise you not to eat sweets before bed because this could create a cycle of bad sleep and increased appetite, which is difficult to break and over time can lead to weight gain, as well as problems such as diabetes.

So now make yourself comfortable, grab that sweet and happy memory, and listen to the rest I must tell you about this sugary subject.

Have you ever wondered what a cake really is and what its origin is?

Certainly, we all have a more or less precise mental image of it, from the cake of childhood to the more composite cakes studied during professional courses.

But although we have a mental image of what a cake is, the talk about this product hides more complexity than you might expect.

The confectionery practice of the Romans began with the art of baking, known after the Hellenic conquest: since then, there were many public ovens so much so that in Rome, in one hundred and sixty-eight B.C. and at the time of Augustus there were about four hundred of them and the guild of "pistores" (bakers) who were slaves from the newly conquered Greece was established.

Until then, the Romans had eaten a cereal puree called "puls", in addition to the cracker, so hard to be used as a dish. The unleavened buns then began to be replaced by loaves of bread, loaves in boxes, sticks made with oil, milk, saffron, rosemary, capers.

In ancient times the first cakes were simple buns made with water and flour to which honey, eggs, spices, butter, cereals, cream, and milk were added, while until recent times "country" cakes were made of bread dough enriched in different ways, from fruit to jam, from liqueurs to spices.

The first news of an elaborate cake is found in the "Satyricon" of Petronius.

Describing the famous banquet of Trimecaine shows us among other delicacies present a square cake in the form of pagan gods. The ingredients, however, both in the case of the Greeks and the Romans, were extremely limited and simple: the cakes were mixed with honey and flour. The sugar, in fact, appeared in Europe only around the eleventh century and in America only after colonization. This precious substance was imported from India by the Arabs.

Cakes have always been used to celebrate moments of "passage" as symbols of prosperity and fertility.

The first elementary sweet preparations were for a long time reserved exclusively for the great solemnities and were often shaped in the shape of animals, as votive offerings to the gods. As history goes on, the available ingredients increase honey, eggs, wheat or oatmeal, milk, and wine and, depending on the geographical area, dried fruit, dates, figs, quinces or cheese.

In the early Middle Ages sweets did not undergo substantial changes, apart from the introduction of the use of essences and distilled perfumes. Within the monasteries, which had preserved the privilege of baking, in addition to the practice of beekeeping and the use of spices, more complex sweets such as waffles and marzipan began to be elaborated.

Until the fifteenth century, the recipe books speak of cookies with an unmistakable oval shape with pointed ends and pancakes, while other sources speak of sugared almonds and some commemorative desserts.

In the seventeenth century, the production of sweets began to spread, first with the packaging of preserves and fruit jellies and then with the inclusion of pastries, such as short pastry, egg and yeast puff pastry, with the addition of cream and cocoa.

At the end of the seventeenth century, in the first laboratory stores, filled cakes made their appearance and at the beginning of the eighteenth century was exposed the oldest of the cakes with butter dough, the Linz or Viennese and at the beginning of the eighteenth century made its appearance the most famous of cakes made with eggs: the Sacher.

During the same century, apothecaries and apothecaries lost the prerogative of the pastry shop; the artisans were able to organize themselves and make the pastry shop a real activity.

A parenthesis should be dedicated to the particular white color of the icing in wedding cakes, which took hold in the nineteenth century and had the function of indicating two concepts: the virgin purity and the richness of the bride. Making the white cake required the use of large quantities of sugar, which was a very expensive commodity, so a very white cake was an indication of great economic resources.

History and culture, after all, have always influenced the taste for cakes, and it can be said that all the greatest cuisines in the world have proposed new recipes.

Cakes that have become famous because they are true masterpieces of refinement and creativity, many of which were created by pastry chefs at the service of a prince or a great reigning house, are now combined with the classic recipes dear to the common man.

Just a few lines ago I mentioned the "Sachertorte", or Sacher cake, and the chocolate rich cake, recognized worldwide as a gastronomic symbol of Austria, Europe, is among the most copied by confectioners, however appreciable the results may be, its recipe is still jealously guarded in Vienna, where it was born.

The question is: who created this legendary cake consisting of two layers of light chocolate paste, with a layer of apricot or cherry jam inside, entirely covered with dark chocolate icing?

We owe the invention of the Sacher cake to the young confectioner Franz Sacher who made it in the one thousand eight hundred and thirty-two in the Austrian capital. Heir to a wealthy family of hoteliers of Jewish origin and a young court baker, it was Chancellor Clemens von Metternich himself who asked him to prepare a cake for a guest, since the official court confectioner was ill. Sacher, then sixteen years old, loved chocolate very much, which he decided to use for his recipe: the result was this extraordinary cake that, legend has it, made Metternich rejoice at the first taste.

Since its invention, the Sacher cake has successfully spread first in Austria, then to the rest of the world. Since the original is protected by a trademark that no one has ever licensed, it can be said that today it is one of the most imitated recipes ever.

After this reference to the Sacher cake, it is impossible not to think of another famous chocolate cake, the beloved Brownie Cake.

There are many stories about the origins of this rich and delicious American cake, but what seems certain is that the official term "Brownie Cake" appeared for the first time in the one thousand eight hundred and ninety-six in a recipe book, in which it was identified as a small chocolate cake made with molasses.

Certain is undoubtedly its American origin and its name derived from the typical brown color. There are those who say that this cake was the result of the work of a careless cook who, in the preparation, forgot to include yeast, others instead speak of a certain Bertha Palmer, famous American businesswoman who lived between one thousand eight hundred and one thousand nine hundred, who asked for a cake that did not dirty her hands and that could be conveniently packaged for a lunch outside the home.

A special mention should of course be reserved for birthday cakes.

Nowadays there are many cultures that celebrate birthdays by lighting candles on the cake and singing the birthday ditty. The number of candles represents the birthday boy's age and usually one must silently make a wish before blowing out the candles.

A theory related to the tradition of candles on the cake originated in ancient Greece. The Greeks created round cakes in honor of Artemis, the goddess of the moon. These cakes were white cakes made of flour and honey and resembled the shape of a satellite. They were lit with candles that represented the glow of the moon and the smoke from the candles carried the prayers of the people to the gods living in the sky. At the end of the celebrations the candles were blown out with a breath to ward off the "evil spirits".

Other scholars believe that the tradition of candles originated in Germany where it was customary to place a candle on the cake as a symbol of the "light of life".

The next time you are celebrating your birthday or the birthday of a friend or relative, you will certainly remember the story of this nice and curious tradition, or you can tell it to all the guests!

One of the cakes that has always been admired and appreciated for its aesthetic component as well as for its taste is undoubtedly the Red Velvet. You want for the color, you want for the texture, has always been a cake that attracts the masses.

Even behind the Red Velvet there is a curious story.

It seems that around the year one thousand nine hundred and forty the Adam Extract Company of Texas was in financial difficulties, like many businesses during the Great Depression, and needed a strategy to see more food coloring.

Mr. Adam and his wife Betty were having lunch at the restaurant at the Waldorf Astoria in New York City (clearly, they weren't in bad shape yet!), when they were served the Red Velvet Cake, colored with beet juice, which had been on the hotel's menu for over a decade.

Adam, once tasted the cake, realized that its red dye could be used to enhance the red color of the cake, without changing the flavor as the beet juice did. So, his company elaborates and produces an original recipe for Red Velvet Cake.

This was nothing more than a chocolate cake, arranged in layers, dyed red with its dye and covered with a milk cream called Ermine Frosting or Original Betty Icing. Later, the latter was replaced by a frosting that did not require baking. They also invented a catchy joke for this cake called "The cake that all wives should bake" (whatever that meant).

It was therefore not an original recipe.

The only thing that made it original was the addition of red color. Because long before the Waldorf started baking the Red Velvet, velvet cakes were quite common.

There was pineapple velvet, lemon velvet and many others. The name Red Velvet Cake was therefore simply referred to a vanilla cake made with red sugar, which was nothing but brown sugar.

And what about cupcakes?

Who has never eaten some cupcakes?

The history of cupcakes begins centuries and centuries ago in America. Already at the end of the eighteenth century the recipe appears in a well-known American cookbook, testimony to its enormous diffusion. Its name probably derives from the way in which they were cooked, that is in cups, hence the use, in the name, of cup, shard, which allowed to save on cooking time. We must consider that the means available to women for cooking, at that time, were not those of today. The cooking was done through wood, so cooking small doses meant to save an enormous amount of time. Beyond this, the use of the cup was probably also useful for measuring the ingredients. The success of these sweets today is mainly due to the TV and their extraordinary and inviting bright color. Especially little girls just cannot resist in front of a cupcake!

Who are the cousins of cupcakes? Well, the Muffins!

Raise your hand if you have never wanted a muffin for breakfast.

Of course, I was joking, stay comfortable and relaxed thinking maybe to enter a cozy pastry shop and be enveloped in a sweet cloud of sugar, to smell the smell of apples baked with cinnamon, cocoa, and cookies.

Let us go back to talking about muffins. This typical English cake, soft like a plum cake, round with a hemispherical cap top and without coating icing, known and appreciated, sees its origins in Victorian England in the eighteenth century.

It was designed by the family bakers of the high society who, initially, prepared it for servitude using stale bread, leftovers of cookies and boiled and mashed potatoes.

The resulting dough was fried and turned into muffins.

Soon all the other social classes also discovered the goodness of this cake that became the favorite for teatime.

The muffins were appreciated to the point that not only were many ovens specialized in their production opened, but the product was also sold on the street by the "Muffin Men" (muffin men) who walked around with wooden trays hanging around their necks, full of muffins. This figure became so important that a lullaby entitled "Oh, do you know the muffin man" was dedicated to him.

Maybe I just managed to make you think of a typical breakfast, well then, we must spend some of our time talking about pancakes.

I realize that I often talk to you about stories of ancient Rome and ancient Greece, but these great civilizations are essential for every culture, history and practice that has been handed down in the centuries to come.

If all roads lead to Rome, all recipes lead to Athens. Yes, you will not believe this, but many of the preparations that we believe we have imported from other continents, such as cheesecake, originate in the time of the Gods of Olympus. That it is because of these almost divine roots that pancakes are so good too? The name recalls its origins and places them in the Anglo-Saxon world, but can you say you really know the history of pancakes?

Yes, the pancake recipe has travelled a long way, crossing continents and entire centuries to the tables all over the world directly from the United States, but the delicious pancakes stuffed with maple syrup, jam, honey or dried fruit were not prepared for the first time in Greece.

In the sixteenth century BC, in fact, Cratino and Magnete, two playwrights' colleagues of the more famous Aristophanes, mention a cake made with water, olive oil and flour, cooked and round, served with honey at breakfast. We can for all intents and purposes say (if only we could taste it!) that it is the ancestor of pancakes, although without yeast.

The question, however, arises spontaneously: how did a sweet Greek pancake turn into a sweet symbol of the Anglo-Saxon world?

As often happened, many Greek traditions and recipes have been assimilated by the Romans. In fact, it is documented that the patricians loved Greek scones enriched with spices.

However, we will have to wait many years for a leavening agent to be introduced in the recipe, but this has not prevented pancakes from spreading throughout Europe and Russia in a form remarkably similar to crepes.

Each country, starting in the Middle Ages, prepared its own variation, some of which have survived to this day as the German Kaiserschmarrn which is cut into small pieces and served with dried fruit and icing sugar.

The success of this simple and versatile dessert also reached, in the same period, the British Isles where the name "pancake" was coined. In fact, we have a trace of it, for the first time, in an official document of the fifteenth century. But, although the name is an English inheritance, the merit of having refined the preparation of the cake to the point of making it look like the pancakes we eat today is all Dutch.

In Holland, in fact, it is a typical and widespread dessert pancakes cooked in a special shaped pan, served one on top of the other, with a sprinkling of powdered sugar.

There is still something missing, however, and those who make pancakes often know it. Nobody in Europe, and until that moment, had added to the recipe a yeast that would give the pancake that soft look that differentiates it from crepes. This is to all intents and purposes an American innovation where the recipe, which draws characteristics from different European variants, crystallizes to become an ambassador of American cuisine.

Have we finished the typical breakfast cakes?
Absolutely not, because if there is something that can invariably accompany our morning drink, it is cookies.

The chocolate chip cookie is the cookie par excellence, at least in the States.

The recipe of round cookies with chocolate chips originates in the thirties of the twentieth century and precisely in Massachusetts. Mrs. Ruth Wakefield used to prepare delicious butter cookies to serve to the customers of her "Toll House Inn", the colonial-style lodge between Boston and New Bedford that she ran with her husband Kenneth. In the process, Ruth realized that she had exhausted a key ingredient in that preparation, Baker's chocolate, a very bitter and melting chocolate that could only be used in baking.

She replaced it with a bar of semi-sweet chocolate, reduced to small pieces, donated to her some time before by her friend Andrew Nestlé. When he took the cookies out of the oven, he noticed that the pieces of chocolate had not melted but were all intact and clearly visible inside the cookies. From the moment he served them in his restaurant, it was a triumph. Ruth's cookie recipe ended up first in the Boston newspaper, then on the radio. From that moment on, there is no American housewife who does not prepare cookies at home, which is served at the "Nestlé Semi-Sweet Chocolate Bar". Andrew Nestlé saw a dizzying increase in the sale of his product and at the time he immediately tried to make the most of it.

In the year one thousand nine hundred and thirty-nine he started producing "chips", or ready-made chocolate chips, and offered Ruth a lifetime supply of chocolate in exchange for permission to print the recipe for "The Famous Toll House Cookie" on the back of his chocolate chip packs. The "chocolate chip cookie" has become not only the quintessence of the stars and stripes confectioner's art, but also the most famous cookie in the world.

Let me take a small step back and return to the sweets that have their origins in ancient Greece, because another dessert, great for a snack or at the end of a meal but maybe less for breakfast, deserves to be mentioned. I am referring to cheesecake.

Cheesecake is one of the most famous and loved desserts in the world.

There are infinite variations, but they all have in common a base made with crumbled dry cookies and butter, a filling of cream cheese and a covering to taste (fruit, chocolate ...).

Typical cake of the Anglo-Saxon world, as the name suggests, but few know the history and origins of the original recipe.

So, let us find out where and how the cheesecake were born.

Many are convinced that the original recipe was born in the United States, but this is not the case.

Historical sources tell of how, already during the Olympics of the eighteenth century seventy-six B.C., the athletes of the island of Delos used to refresh themselves with a cake made with honey and sheep's cheese, an energetic and caloric meal.

Callimachus also tells that in the same period - eighth century BC - in Greece lived Egimius, a man who had dedicated his time to writing a manual in which he explained the art of making cheesecakes.

Later the Romans modified the recipe, creating a cake with two discs of dough with sweet cheese in the middle, this is how Cato the Censor describes it in his work "De Agri Culture".

Little is known about how cheesecake has been handed down from the ancient world to the modern one.

Surely the expansion of the Roman Empire made the recipe spread all over Europe.

But when does it appear in America?

The modern version of the cheesecake, with crispy base and cream cheese, was born in Philadelphia in one thousand eight hundred and seventy-two, by the dairy producer James L. Kraft.

The milkman, trying to reproduce the famous French cheese Neufchatel, obtained an equally tasty cream cheese, which later became famous all over the world under the name of Philadelphia.

This spreadable cheese became the main ingredient of modern cheesecake, which spread quickly in the United States and the Anglo-Saxon world.

Today cheesecake is widespread all over the world, in many variations: cooked and not, sweet, and salty, with and without icing.

The famous New York cheesecake, for example, is baked in the oven and uses sugar, eggs, and milk cream for the filling.

It is also characterized by a glaze made with sour cream, vanilla seeds, and icing sugar, which, after browning in the oven, is topped with chocolate chips or fruit.

In Asia, instead, typical local ingredients are used, such as matcha tea powder, milk, mango, and ginger.

In Europe there are endless versions: from the cheesecake to the Baileys typical of Ireland, to the one with the skyr cheese typical of Iceland, passing through the Polish cheesecake made with twarog cheese and raisins.

Another very American dessert is the banana split.

It is a cake that involves a long cut banana that is covered with ice cream, melted chocolate or other topping and, if you like, also nuts, fresh fruit, whipped cream or other.

How not to appreciate the perfect balance between a fruit course and a dessert? A delicious and energetic snack for children and teens. The banana split is undoubtedly a simple and delicious invention that has not ceased to be a world-wide success. But who invented this dessert?

It may seem excessive to you to speak of a real "invention", referring to the banana split, and yet the dish has been the subject of a patent.

Its story, which cloaks itself in legend, begins at the beginning of the Twentieth Century in Boston. Here, an anonymous travelling ice-cream vendor would split a banana with the whole peel and fill it with chocolate ice cream. Who immediately understood the potential for success of the banana split was a student at the University of Pittsburgh who worked in his family's bar in Latrobe, Pennsylvania: it was David Evans Strickler. He patented the dessert, with a variant: the peeled banana.

In Latrobe, the centenary of the invention of the split banana was celebrated; a tribute to this joy of the palate, but also to its inventor who, without any doubt by the inhabitants of the city, was David Evans Strickler.

The inhabitants of Wilmington, Ohio, on the other hand, have some doubts. According to their version of the story of the origins of the banana split, it was the year one thousand nine hundred and seven when Ernest Hazard asked the employees of his restaurant for some new ideas to refresh the dessert menu. No one was able to provide him with a fairly innovative idea. So, he decided to do it himself: he cut the pulp of a banana and filled it with ice cream.

After all this talk about extraordinary sweets I hope you did not feel like going to the kitchen for a snack. This is not the time, trust me.

Save your appetite for breakfast tomorrow morning, maybe you could enjoy a special breakfast tomorrow, for example if you stop at the usual place to rush to get a muffin and coffee you will smile thinking about Victorian England of the eighteenth century, or next time you make pancakes for yourself or for the whole family or friends you can tell how the Greeks invented the ancestors of pancakes.

Making a cake for others is good for your mental health, baking it for yourself is a form of awareness.

When baking sweets for others, it can also be a useful way to communicate your feelings. Several studies reveal that donating food created with one's own hands, in this case a cake, can be useful for people who have difficulty expressing what they feel through words. It is no coincidence that many cultures view food as an expression of love. Donating it is even more so.

Baking requires a lot of attention. You have to weigh, calculate, concentrate physically to roll out the dough. If you focus on smell and taste, you are present with what you are creating, creating an act of awareness of the present moment that can help reduce stress a bit like meditation.

Numerous scientific papers link creative expression to general well-being. Whether it is painting or making music or cooking, people experience a feeling of stress relief.

Finally, the mind takes over that particular mechanism of searching for lost time, that dazzling reference to distant memories, mostly linked to childhood memories or happy events.

Grab that moment of joy that one of the sweets whose history we have known during the previous pages has brought you back and hold on to it.

Enjoy the feeling of lightheartedness that unravels in your soul and with it begins to slip into your deepest sleep.

Feel good as that child who had no thoughts at all, feel like that child on his birthday, imagine going back to the kitchen of his childhood home to bake cookies with chocolate chips.

Imagine being able to enter a magical pastry shop, all decorated with pastel colors such as pink, light blue and cream, and you can admire beautiful shop windows of colored sweets as in the movies of yesteryear.

Inhale imagining the scent of that pastry shop, a warm and enveloping scent that smells of home and moments of joy.

Often children are saddened by having to leave the places where they are having fun, well, even adults.

And you know what the good news is? That you will never be sent away from here.

In this magical place you can stay whenever you want, sink into a soft armchair, and relax as if you were swimming in a sea of cream.

Wouldn't it be nice to sleep on a cloud of cream?
Soft, soft, smelling of sugar and vanilla.

Sit on your personal cloud and let yourself go.

Do not think about anything, just how good you feel on a cloud of cream.

Tomorrow morning you will feel regenerated and a better person, and when you want to, you can always climb on your cloud of cream and relax, or take back that happy thought, the image of that magnificent cake on which you blew the candles.

Now let yourself be rocked by the cloud of cream.

Feel that with your legs, back and shoulders you are pleasantly sinking into the cream cloud.

Breathe, relax, let your body become as soft as the delicious, melted toppings over desserts.

It is okay, trust me. Here it is a perfect and safe world.

You will dream of cakes and confetti tonight, of colorful cupcakes and soft muffins. Soft as the pillow where you are about to fall asleep.

You have a cream mattress and a muffin pillow.

You are so sleepy, and you have all the time and everything you need to sleep blissfully.

Let yourself go, let yourself fall asleep with the sweetness of cream.

You are surrounded by sweetness, a sweetness to your favorite tastes.

Sweet dreams.

Chapter 7 Feel Like A Fish

Hey, hello!

How are you?

I hope everything is going great, but if not, do not worry, you have come to the right place to recover your strength and energy.

Together we will let all the worries that grieve you sink into the profundity of the ocean.

We will let all the anxieties and worries that you carry on you like a ballast go out to sea carried by the currents.

The important thing is that you are mentally settled to get on a beautiful boat with me and be ready to let go.

Make yourself comfortable, lower the back of the seat as when you are on an airplane or tuck yourself under the covers. Make sure that you have time, space, and warmth, that you don't need to get up to go to the bathroom or to say good night to those who live with you.

Turn off everything you do not need and eliminate all forms of distraction.

Take me by the hand and let's go.

Did you know that watching fish is a healthy pastime?
Seeing them swimming and wandering around, underwater or in an aquarium, is hypnotic and relaxing, calms the heartbeat and lowers the pressure.

Yes, aquariums are an oasis of calm and relaxation in these times of hectic and stressful work and urban life.
You can also learn from the fish to slow down and relax.

It has now been proven that watching fish swim in an aquarium is not only good for your health, but also good for your health!

According to the researchers, the benefits are proportional to the number of fish and the quality of observation: the more fish in the aquarium, the more the person is captivated by their movements, the more positive effects can be achieved both physically and mentally.

This is certainly not the first study to show how natural environments and animals themselves can bring well-being into everyone's life: disconnecting the mind from work and everyday problems has become a fundamental need for everyone.

Standing in front of an aquarium staring at the vaulting of fish is a fascinating vision that allows our brain to fully immerse itself and not think about anything but the wanderings of our friends.

This relaxing effect is remarkably like that of meditation.

The importance of observing nature, especially animals, seems to be deeply rooted in the human psyche, experts say. The understanding and appreciation by humans for the natural world, and our preference for natural environments, could be the product of biological evolution.

Getting lost watching the fish swim with great beauty, without predictability, attracts our attention and induces us to relax. So, even if the dog has always been man's best friend, we should not exclude a friend with fins!

Of course, not all of us can afford to have an aquarium at home, as for all creatures in the world to take care of it requires time, passion, patience, space, of course even money is obvious, and much more that I'm not going to list.

Yet, all of us, regardless of where, how, when, who we are and what we do, have access to an exceptional and super powerful power: imagination.

So now, as always, let go and start imagining that you have the most beautiful aquarium in the world, or the aquarium you would like to have and that you could make appear if you had a magic wand.

Have you done it?

That is great! Now we can start observing the magical world of fish and find out more about them.

The first fish I want to tell you about is the Guppy, also known as million fish and rainbow fish, is one of the most popular and easy to manage in the aquarium. Nice, with fascinating shapes and colors, it is robust and adaptable to various habitats.

The Guppy fish is native to South America and is called "million fish" because of its enormous and easy profilins, a characteristic that has allowed its breeding and genetic selection since the early twentieth century.

With its red and blue, fluorescent bands then there is the Neon Fish, which offers an extraordinary spectacle in any aquarium. It is a small freshwater fish native to the Amazon that loves to live exclusively in groups.

I could list you many types of fish, but instead of a storyteller you could mistake me for an aquarium salesclerk, so let's get back to us and our imagination.

From the moment everything is possible in our imagination, what do you say to dive into the giant aquarium?

Don't worry, you don't need to equip yourself with oxygen tanks and other instruments, you can imagine you are in a diver's suit or why not in a comfortable and very dry bubble.

What is great is that you can enjoy the soothing oil from the water.

There is no gravity, there is no internet connection, there is no network, there is no way that someone will come to fish for you.

All sounds of the chaotic outside world are cut off, muffled under liters and liters of clear water, water that envelops you and protects you in its world full of nice, elegant, and colorful fish.

Since ours is an aquarium of pure and bizarre fantasy, which does not follow any rules that we would otherwise have to follow scrupulously so as not to risk compromising the health of our finned friends, we do not have to worry about whether the fish inside are fresh or salt water, whether they live together in peace or not, whether they are male or female, and so on. We pretend we are in the middle of the ocean or in a huge lake if it is better.

Imagine that you are circling slowly in the depths and while you are intent on looking one by one at the numerous fins nobilis scattered on the seabed, those species of giant mussels that populate the Mediterranean, suddenly you stop to observe a form of motionless cut, a short, fast, and continuous swaying at the top of the figure, like short and thick vibrating lashes. Strange, do you think, what kind of fish is this?

And then you approach slowly, but from above you still do not understand... Don't worry, all you have to do is to change your view, leaning gently to the side, and suddenly out of nowhere an unmistakable, two-dimensional shape appears to you, is a fish that you would never expect to see there: a St. Peter's fish.

The origin of the name St. Peter's fish is linked to a legend according to which the dark spots on its sides are the footprints of the apostle Peter who allegedly grabbed the fish at Christ's request to extract a gold coin from its mouth. The contact with the hands of the Saint made the fish's fingerprints remain in a black spot that he transmitted to his descendants. Other popular traditions instead indicate that this is the fish that Jesus multiplied on the Lake of Tiberias, and that the two black spots on the belly are the footprints of Jesus, left when he took the fish in his hands, before the multiplication. Scientifically it is called

Zeus, which means Jupiter because the fish was consecrated to the King of the Gods.

Among the various fish that I want you to imagine now to meet is the Betta Splendens, better known as Siamese fighting fish.

If you were to take a five- or six-year-old boy to a tropical fish store to have him observe the tanks and then ask him which is his favorite fish, if among the various guests there is at least one Betta Splendens, with long red or blue veil fins swaying in midwater, you can bet he will show you just that. It's hard not to be charmed by this little friend with fins that surpasses all other freshwater fish in terms of variety of colors and shapes of the fin, which has been the subject of countless studies on behavioral analysis of animals and that better than many others is suitable to live even in the small spaces of home aquariums.

The history of this fish, scattered with surprising events, is an extraordinary testimony to the life force of nature and the infinite possibilities of evolution, but it is also proof of the power of human passion when it acts in tune with nature.

This is the secret of the small but wonderful little fish watching you from behind the glass, swaying haughty and silent with tight lips.

It is in those tight lips that the first trace of the origin of this fish hides, like all fish that adopt gill breathing, but swim with their mouths closed. It is not for demeanor, as one might think knowing his character, but because the Betta does not breathe only through the gills, which he has anyway, but through the labyrinth: an organ that develops during the first month of life and allows him to breathe, emerge on the surface and breathe plenty of air mouth. To learn more about this prodigious organ we must go back in our minds to about four hundred million years ago. Our planet has already existed for at least four billion years, but no animal has ever laid its paws on its surface. The lands that emerged are still grouped in large continents close together, which have only the semblance of today's continents. Geological activity is extremely high, but the first forests are already forming and the conditions for animal life outside the water are maturing. At first insects appear, but the actual animal life still takes place underwater: it is the age of the fish.

The temperature of the seas is high. Probably there is no ice and in this "tropical" climate the progressive colonization of the mainland by plants generates semi-earthly habitats rich in sediments and nutrients, swamps, river estuaries where life literally explodes replacing the simple and primitive algae, which already exist for three billion years.

While the first terrestrial animals appear, other fish take a different evolutionary path: they do not develop lungs, but a simpler respiratory organ called a labyrinth, collected in a small space between the gills and the mouth. This special organ allows them to breathe even in the air, out of the water, their natural element.

The branch fed by labyrinthine is less prosperous and gives different benefits. These fish maintain an exceedingly small size, but specialize in living in extremely protected areas, often richer in plants than water. Over millions of years, they overcome the catastrophic wave of Cretaceous extinction that wipes large reptiles off the face of the earth and continue to differentiate themselves into numerous families and species to this day. Some of these fish colonize the waterways of Indochina, from Siam (today's Thailand) to Malaysia, progressively differentiating themselves in more than 50 species that today are called Betta and developing the territorial, combative nature of an animal accustomed to living in small spaces and the ability to jump out of the water to move from one pool to another when space becomes insufficient.

The evolutionary branch of labyrinthine does not express all this potential, but, in a certain sense, develops it within itself for millions of years, and then manifests it between the end of the nineteenth and the end of the twentieth century, when the breeding by man gives life to the whirling development of shapes and colors that can be observed today in aquariums around the world that host Betta splendens.

It is difficult to say with precision when man began to breed Betta splendens. There are no certain documents until the nineteenth century, but the first evidence suggests that at that time these fish were already bred in Siam for generations, probably hundreds of years. Some archives in the Sukhotai region, dating back to the fourteenth century, speak of fish farming for fighting purposes. For the first Westerners to observe them in the 19th century, they are the "fighting fish of Siam". The Thai people instead call them "pla kat", literally "biting fish".

When the King of Thailand Rama III decided to make a gift of these fish to Westerners in the nineteenth and forties, the breeding of these fish is obviously already mature and consolidated, but it certainly did not begin for ornamental purposes. Being "biting fish", fighting fish, and for a long time, perhaps until a few years before the reign of Rama III, the main purpose of their breeding was fighting. According to the mainly oral tradition handed down in Thailand, the "biting fish" were already known at least six hundred years ago. We can imagine that, initially, catching fighting fish in small streams, ponds or irrigation channels of rice paddies were a pastime for children. The fish could then be put in a pot and made to fight. From here to breed them, the pace must have been rather rapid: they are robust, accustomed to small spaces and for territorial instinct, competitive and prone to mating, even in captivity. In the rural areas of Siam, therefore, the idea of breeding these fish to select the most suitable for fighting must have been progressively born, handing down through the generations the methods to train and select them. We know that progressively, fish fighting as a simple pastime has taken on the character of a traditional art and has become an opportunity for real competitions, accompanied by bets or cash prizes.

To date it is reasonable to think that even in the farms of fighting fish there were occasionally mutations that gave rise to different fish, with interesting fins: caudal longer than normal, bizarre colors. Breeders must have noticed these characters and kept them in the following generations, for pure aesthetic pleasure, maybe to show these fish at home, in glass jars instead of terracotta, or to involve in their passion also children and women, excluded from fighting competitions but surely inclined to appreciate the beauty of the little Bettas with longer and more colorful fins than usual.

The United States is undoubtedly currently the second home of the Betta splendens. Already in the immediate postwar period, you could buy Betta splendens for breeding in your home aquarium. They are already very well developed and rounded fish with long, caudal fins. The small Bettas reproduce easily - intensive Thai breeding has enhanced this feature - and the American breeders, who have no interest in fighting, but a large market of aquarium enthusiasts, choose to aim for the selection of the best colors and fins. In just a few years, the genetic potential of these labyrinthine, which had been hatching for millions of years, exploded. Between the 1950s and 1960s, several American breeders established the character of the Betta veil tail, with its exceptionally long veiled caudal fin. The veil tails are reimported back into the prolific Thai farms and from there they spread all over the world.

Moving from a small fish to a very large one, I thought that maybe up close it might even have something scary, but certainly one of the most fascinating fish to admire in a giant aquarium could be the swordfish.

Can I perhaps fail to mention origins that sink in ancient Greece?

It is said that the Myrmidons, wanting to avenge the killing of Achilles, attacked the Trojans.

The Myrmidons are a people of Greek mythology, descended from Myrmidon, son of Zeus.

They were an ancient people of Thessaly of which Achilles was king and that he led with him, in large numbers, to the Trojan war. According to a tradition, the people took their name from their king Myrmidon, son of Zeus and Eurimedusa, whom the god had seduced by assuming the appearance of an ant. Myrmidons are also mentioned by Homer in the Iliad, where their blind obedience to the orders of Achilles in the Trojan War is painted: they often obeyed even in a very cold and cruel way, just to show their nature as "former ants". In the Iliad five Myrmidon heads are mentioned: Alcimedon, Eudorus, Phoenix, Menoetius and Pisander.

The Trojans, to avoid reprisal, escaped and then the Myrmidons, angry for not having reached the intent, let themselves drown. In order to pass on this noble gesture Tethys, sea goddess, turned them into fish with a long rostrum in memory of their weapon.

Because of this legend, still today in the South of Italy, the swordfish fishing takes place following a precise procedure, the fishermen, on traditional boats for such fishing, establish a sort of dialogue when they spot the fish, exclusively in Greek. When the boat is near the swordfish, it is an absolute tradition that the sailor "speaks" to the fish.

Now that we have talked about small fish and big fish, why not go, and have a look in the fish paradise?

I am talking of course about the fabulous reef!

The Great Barrier Reef is located off the east coast of Australia.

It is very extensive, and it is the only one in the world, which is why it is essential to protect it, or rather it would be better to say vital, because if it were to disappear all the colorful fish and its extraordinary sea creatures that populate it would disappear and become extinct forever.

The Great Barrier was discovered by Captain James Cook in the eighteenth century during a voyage in the southern hemisphere. Before Cook's arrival, the Wall was known only to a few local indigenous tribes, the Aborigines. Today the Reef is well known and appreciated especially by snorkeling tourists, who can see with their own eyes' clownfish, colorful fish, stingrays, sharks, beautiful corals, mollusks, and sea turtles that can live up to over one hundred twenty years.

Declared a World Heritage Site in the year one thousand nine hundred and eighty-one, it also became an Australian National Heritage Site in the year two thousand and seven. The Great Barrier Reef is protected and safeguarded to limit the impact of human intervention in relation to fishing and tourism. Some areas are particularly protected, because of their fragility they have been banned from fishing and underwater tourism, in order to protect the sea creatures that populate it such as dugongs, whales and green turtles.

Coral reefs have a strategic function of protecting the population that populates the mainland from storms and waves that could hit the coasts and sweep away entire villages, acting as a protective cushion between the sea and man.

Climate change, fishing, pollution, and the hostile creatures that inhabit it are the main sources of threat to the health of the reef. Other hazards could be accidents between boats, oil spills, but also powerful tropical cyclones.

Do you know what the bright colors of corals come from? From algae. Moreover, only colored corals are alive, white ones are dead.

Speaking about corals, I know an ancient story related to the Great Barrier Reef, and I want to tell it to you now that you are comfortable and immersed in the depths of the sea.

This is the Legend of Pania, the Maiden of the Barrier Reef.

Pania was a beautiful maiden who lived in the sea on the east coast of the North Island of New Zealand. During the day she would swim with the creatures of her world, the coral reef, but after sunset she would reach a stream that flowed into the bay where the city of Napier now exists. She would swim up the stream to an area where she could rest among the linen bushes.

Karitoki, the beautiful son of a Maori chief, quenched his thirst every evening with the sweet water of the stream where Pania went to rest. He did not realize that she had been watching him for many weeks until one night she whispered a spell that the wind brought to Karitoki, who turned and saw Pania emerge from her hiding place.

Karitoki had never seen such a beautiful girl and fell in love with her instantly. Pania fell in love too; they exchanged their vows to each other and got married in secret. They went to Karitoki's house, but it was dark, and no one saw them enter. When the sun rose, Pania prepared to leave but Karitoki tried to stop her. She explained to him that being a sea creature, every morning the sirens called her, and she had to reach them because otherwise she would die. She promised to return to him every night and their marriage continued in this way.

Karitoki bragged to friends describing to them the beauty of his wife, but no one believed him because they had never seen her. Frustrated, Karitoki consulted a kaumatua (wise old man) from the village who believed Karitoki's story because he knew the existence of the ocean maidens. The kaumatua told Karitoki that as a sea creature, Pania would not be allowed to return to the sea if she ate cooked food.

That night, while Pania was sleeping, Karitoki took a bite of cooked food and put it in her mouth. At that moment, the Ruru owl started bubbling so loudly that Pania woke up. Horrified by Karitoki's behavior that had endangered her life, Pania fled the house and ran to the sea. Her people emerged and carried her down into the depths as Karitoki swam frantically into the ocean to find her. He never saw her again.

Even today some people say that when they look into the deep waters beyond the coral reef, they can see Pania with her arms outstretched as if she was calling her lover even though they cannot tell if she is begging Karitoki to explain his gesture, or if she is simply expressing her love for him.

Napier's sea is now protected by Moromore, the son of Pania and Karitoki. He is the Kaitiaki (guardian) of the area, a taniwha (spirit) who often disguises himself as a shark, parsnip, or octopus.

Pania, often called "Pania of the Barrier Reef", is a mythological Māori figure, and a symbol of the city of Napier in New Zealand.

On June the tenth one thousand nine hundred and fifty-four along the Marine Parade, the Napier waterfront, the then New Zealand Prime Minister Sidney Holland inaugurated a statue dedicated to Pania, which has since become a tourist destination.

The statue has often been compared to the Little Mermaid statue in Copenhagen; there is a similarity between the two figures, both statues are small, in bronze, and near the sea, and both are based on similar stories.

Having just mentioned the little mermaid protagonist of one of the most famous and appreciated childhood fairy tales, how can we not stop for a few moments to imagine that during our swim we meet one of these mythical creatures?

Whether we are adults or children, we would all like to see a real mermaid. They are beautiful sea creatures, half human, and half sea creatures, and since everything in our soothing journey into the abyss is possible, we can imagine that our dry air bubble leads us, after the Great Barrier Reef where we met Pania, to deep depths where we are enchanted by these enchanting creatures.

Let us surrender to the hypnosis that the sirens exerted on Ulysses, as told in the Odyssey, and in the meantime, we discover something curious about them.

In Hellenic mythology the Sirens are the daughters of the god of the rivers Achelous born from the drops of blood that came out of the wounds caused by Hercules (or Heracles) when he broke his horn.

Their appearance was completely different from how it is presented to us now in many books of myths and legends.

The Sirens were in fact half woman and half bird and not as one would expect half woman and half fish.

Mermaids are conventionally depicted as beautiful girls with long golden hair and flowing hair, with a long fishtail instead of legs. Sometimes they are associated with dangerous events such as storms and drownings, while in other popular traditions (or sometimes within the same tradition), they are gentle and benevolent creatures, offering gifts or falling in love with human beings.

Probably the transformation of the Siren from woman-bird to woman-fish occurred during the second century AD. There are presumably two reasons for this mutation.

The first reason may derive from the fact that an amanuensis of the time, in some bestiary, mistakenly wrote the Latin word "pennis" instead writing "pinnis" which means fin. Another reason could derive from the spread of Christianity that saw these creatures as evil beings.

Since only angels could have attributes such as wings, it was decided to change them into fins.

The Sirens were for many centuries considered creatures of the evil, evil and a symbol of perdition. Only with Homer was their figure ennobled and they became charitable creatures and companions of souls in the world beyond.

After the "dark" period of Christianity, considered to be evil beings again, the Sirens, with Andersen's fable, found again the reputation as compassionate beings and symbol of tragic love.

The ancient Northerners said that just outside the water, mermaids could become women, but as soon as they returned to the water, they became mermaids again. According to them, mermaids would have exceptionally long hair and strange colors, to make them confuse with algae. From their hair would come out brilliant, gems, pearls, and precious stones. All mermaids would have human teeth, but behind them they would also have one or two rows of sharp and thin teeth, which they use to trap and chew fish and to chop algae (but for some of them they are also used to chew sailor meat). They would have hands with webbed fingernails and fingers. Needless to say, mermaids don't wear bras or clothes - although they are often imagined like that - because they get into trouble in the water, but they love to adorn themselves with algae or shells.

In more recent times compared to antiquity, however, the sirens did not enjoy a good reputation, on the contrary, it was thought that they brought bad luck if encountered in the open sea by sailors at sea.

About it is told in a legend...

Once upon a time there was a boat of fishermen, who had gone too far out to sea because of the strong wind. As they reached beyond the imposing and menacing cliffs of Moher, in the lush green Ireland, they felt lost and the sight of a mermaid sitting on a rock emphasized their fears. They tried to get away, but the siren continued to follow them singing a melancholy love song. And the more she sang the louder the wind blew, and the more she cried the more the waves rose high.

The captain, a man of great experience, after a short time understood what was happening and gathered his sailors on deck to explain the situation to them.

"This mermaid must be in love with a sailor in the crew, that's why she doesn't want to let us go and is so desperate. She is sick with love"

The sailors looked at each other incredulously trying to understand who the object of the attention and love of the young creature had been. Failing to reach a conclusion, they decided to draw lots to see who would stop to console the siren to allow the rest of the crew to return home safe and sound.

Sean, a handsome young man with long coppery hair, was extracted. He was a strong man, intelligent and useful to the crew because he knew how to steer a ship even in the absence of the Captain. To lose him would have been a great damage...

So, the Captain decided to give them a second chance: they would repeat the draw the next day. The situation did not improve, on the contrary the storm was getting stronger and stronger, it had also started raining and lightning in the distance were tearing the sky. The draw was made again, but Sean's name was always the first to come out.

The Captain, stubborn, gave him a third chance, but again, on the third day, it was always Sean's name that came out first. Now it was no longer possible to wait and the sailors were exhausted and desperate and began to hate that young man who was leading them to death, not understanding why the Captain's attentions towards him.

"It's only fair that I go," Sean began, standing up.

"Three times my name has come out, fate wants me to console the young mermaid. Leave me with her alone for a while".

So, he went out on the bridge, headed aft and straight towards the mermaid and sang a song from his childhood, and as he sang, the storm was moving away, the thunder was getting further and further away, and the wind began to calm down. The siren stopped sobbing and the sea calmed down with her. Their voices touched each other for long moments, as if their souls touched each other.

But they could not stay, he had to go... And the siren understood.

A ray of sunshine came out of the black clouds and the ship was able to resume its journey home, far from the rocks, far from death.

After that adventure, Sean took the place of the old Captain and sailed all his life with skill and righteousness, without ever having an accident, always coming out unharmed from every storm. But, after meeting the siren, he never sang again.

Ireland is an island and, as such, could not fail to be attracted by the charm of mermaids.

There are many creatures connected with the underwater world, for example even the Banshee that dwelt, according to folklore, near springs and streams, they with human features, the others with a body half human and fish.

In neighboring Scotland is even told of the Kelpie, fairy horses that dwelt in springs and streams, often represented both with the appearance of normal equines, and with fish tails.

According to other ancient Irish legends, the Banshee were visible only to those who were close to death and not always had benevolent connotations, on the contrary, they were often considered as real witches.

Let us stay in Ireland because in the land of dark beer is famous the legend of another mermaid, a creature called Li Ban, the "holy mermaid". Li Ban, young daughter of a King, found herself transformed into an immortal mermaid, with a salmon tail, due to a flood. After three hundred years the monks found the mermaid and baptized her according to the Christian ritual. One of the monks offered her a choice: live for another three hundred years or die to be immediately beatified. Li Ban sacrificed her immortality to ascend to heaven.

In nearby Cornwall, the figure of the mermaid was also used to illustrate the two natures of Christ. While the mermaid was human and fish, so Jesus could be both human and divine, a message that would strike the inhabitants of this isolated region whose lives were intertwined with the sea. From generation to generation, the legend of the Zennor siren is passed down in those places of the sea, according to which the song of a church choirman named Mathew Trewhella is said to have lured a siren ashore from the depths of the sea. According to the story, every Sunday she sat at the back of the church, enchanted by his beautiful voice. One day, no longer containing her infatuation, she took him to the small stream that still flows through the center of the village and leads into the sea at Cove Pendour nearby. Mathew Trewhella was never seen again. On warm summer evenings, walking in the picturesque cove now called "Mermaid Cove", it is said that the two lovers can be heard singing happily together, and their voices can be heard through the roar of the crashing waves.

Another legend about a European mermaid is related to the city of Warsaw. It is said that a long time ago there were two sirens, sisters among them, swimming from their home in the abysses, to the shores of the Baltic Sea. They were incredibly beautiful creatures even though they had fish tails instead of legs. One of them decided to swim away towards the Denmark Strait and today you can admire her sitting on a rock at the entrance to the port of Copenhagen. The other one swam to the coastal city of Gdansk and from there continued up the Vistula River. Probably right at the foot of what is today the Old Town is the place where she came out of the water to rest on the sandy shore and she liked the place so much that she decided to settle down. The fishermen who lived in the area soon realized that when they were fishing, someone would shake the river waters, tangling the nets and releasing the fish that were caught in them. So they decided to hunt down the culprit and put an end to these damages once and for all; but when they heard the siren song, they fell in love with it, giving up their intentions. From that moment on, the mermaid entertained the fishermen every night with her wonderful songs, until one day a rich merchant, walking along the riverbank, laid his eyes on the fascinating creature. He immediately thought that if he caught her, he could earn a lot of money by showing her at fairs. The merchant quickly put his evil plan into action: with a trick he captured the mermaid and locked her up in a wooden shack without access to water. The cries of the beautiful woman-fish came to a young laborer, son of a fisherman, who with the help of a friend managed to free her one night. The mermaid, grateful for the help received from the inhabitants of the town, promised that if they were ever in danger, she would come back to protect them.

After so much talk about pretty and enchanting sirens, you may be surprised to learn that there are also bad sirens. Yeah, some legends want as protagonists these creatures with a truly rebellious character.

Among the evil mermaids we find for example Orejona; Orejona is a mermaid with amphibious characteristics: she has women's legs, but webbed hands and gills. Orejona is an alien mermaid, descended from a golden ship and then landed in Lake Titicaca. In the sea caves often live beautiful mermaids like her but equally cruel and ruthless, in fact they love to eat human flesh and cover their cave with skulls in which the souls of drowned sailors are locked.

The Ningyo instead are sirens of Japan, very shy and harmless.
In Thailand lives the Duyugun, a siren with long hair. They are not attractive and the first of them is said to be a very naughty little girl transformed by the spirits into a mermaid, as if she were a recurring punishment.
In the delta of the Niger River in Nigeria, Afriga, lives Mami Wata a mermaid who gives magical powers to those who see her.

In the Red Sea there are mermaids who, according to legend, are the daughters of Pharaoh Ramses' soldiers, drowned and then married to mermaids.

Well, if I wanted, I could stay and tell you about other sirens around the world, but I don't want you to fall asleep out of boredom and exhaustion. I just want you to relax and enjoy the pleasant entertainment that these stories can convey.

As we have seen anyway, in every place there is a legend, and in every respectable sea place, very often the protagonist of this legend is a mermaid.

Now, why don't you let yourself go like those sailors to the hypnotic singing of the sweet sirens?

Make yourself as comfortable as a sailor lying in the sun on the deck of his ship.

Enjoy the oblivion offered by the rhythmic rocking of the sea and the beauty offered by the creatures that populate it.

Let the abysses silence the whole world that often deafen us, listen only to the sirens' song.

Swim with your bubble in the crystal-clear waters amidst the vibrant and fragile creatures of uncontaminated beauty.

You are in a wonderful place, you are safe.

You can stay whenever you want.

Relax and let yourself go.

You are like a sea creature too, light and at ease in the currents of the Reef.

You can fall asleep among colorful fish and enchanting creatures, among long and sinuous fins.

You are part of the marine kingdom now.

Let yourself go to blue dreams.

Swim in your sleep, it will be an enchanted sleep.

Chapter 8 Turn Page

How many times would we like to move on?

It would be easy, no?

Turn the page and leave the bad things in the previous chapter, so that we can start a new one.

Well, it is not easy. It is not easy for anyone, not even superheroes.

So, do you know how we can do it?

We can really turn the page starting from dedicating time to ourselves and prepare to enjoy a beautiful and healthy dose of deep sleep.

Often, we dedicate ourselves to reading before sleeping, and in that gesture, is enclosed for many a ritual that can prove to be a real panacea, that is: sniffing the smell of paper.

Raise your hand to those who never happened to smell a new book, or even an old one, if linked to particular memories. I doubt that it has not happened at least once.

I am a serial book sniffer, but I do not miss magazines with smooth and glossy pages, the ones that give off a great smell.

I avoid sniffing outdated books, those of at least twenty years to understand us, because the risk is to inhale unpleasant and quite dangerous mold, especially if these books have passed through several different hands and places.

Having a book in our hands, perhaps one of our favorites, leads us to live it with all the senses. If we cannot taste it, at least we do not just read it. We have to touch it, flip through it and listen to the soft noise of the pages, look at its and... smell it.

What is the smell that emanates from books? A mixture of everything that comes from paper, ink, and glue.

There is no doubt that the smell of some books is intimately linked to those who have owned them, this is a different aspect but no less important. Some books bring back certain memories because something of the person who handled them gets caught between the pages. Is it just suggestion? Who knows?

The book has this power to absorb something of the reader.

That smell, incredibly special scent associated with mystery, inexplicable, often conveys the feeling of being in a special place.

When you enter any bookstore, it is almost inevitable to associate that scent with one of the most beautiful moments of our life, such as the first years of school.

The smell of paper evokes attention, love, a sense of belonging, the possibility of discovering wonderful worlds. Of course, there is a reaction related to neurotransmitters and neuronal circuits, but it's nice to think that the smell of books is related to magic.

And what immediately comes to mind with the books and the smell of books?

The silence.

The quiet.

The feeling of peace and culture that only very few places in the world can convey, such as museums, places of worship, but above all: libraries.

Imagine being able to enter a library and enjoy the silence offered by the environment, where everything is muffled by paper and the only noises allowed are those of the caressing rustling of the pages.

Libraries are fascinating places, so quiet and full of knowledge. Even those who do not read are usually impressed when they see so many books collected in one room.

Libraries have always contained the knowledge of humanity. Often, to carry out this honorable task, beautiful buildings have been built, which would make hundreds or thousands of books at home.

Do you want to know the history of some of the oldest libraries in the world?

Follow me, tilt the back of the armchair, or crumple the cushion a little bit to settle better, and let yourself be carried away.

In two thousand and sixteen the oldest university in the world - the University of Fez, Morocco - reopened its doors to the public after an extensive renovation project. Within its walls there is a fabulous and ancient Islamic library. The library opened its doors in the nineteenth and fifties nineteen hundred A.D., and to this day it has been used by scholars for over a millennium - becoming part of the oldest libraries in the world.

It was an erudite woman named Fatima who founded the University and built the mosque, the library and the school associated with it. It was the time when Algebra was being born. Her diploma, written on a wooden tablet, is on display today at the University. Among the many ancient manuscripts that the library has restored are an original manuscript for the ancient Islamic legal system, and a ninth century Koran - the oldest work in the entire collection.

The Vatican is home to one of the oldest libraries in Europe, formally recognized in the fifteenth century seventy-five - even though it had actually been operating long before. From the fourth century, in fact, there is evidence in the Vatican of an archiving system for manuscripts and other important documents, while the figure of the librarian appeared from the eighth century.

In the mid-fifteenth century Pope Nicholas V decided that the proliferation of manuscripts in Latin, Greek and Hebrew should be made available for scholars to read and study. The Library was built inside the Vatican Palace, with an entrance through the Belvedere Courtyard.

Then, one of the richest and oldest libraries in Europe is located in the Portuguese University of Coimbra. King João 5th - from which the building takes its name - had the library built under his patronage between one thousand seven hundred and seventeen and one thousand seven hundred and twenty-eight. The baroque style library was decorated by the best artists in Portugal and is wonderful.

The University of Salamanca, in nearby Spain, was created at the behest of King Alfonso the Ninth of Leon in the year one thousand two hundred and eighteen. In the one thousand two hundred fifty-four, the Magna Carta of Alfonso the Tenth listed the role of "Estacionario", the owner of a "station" of books, which was paid by the University to keep copies of the works for consultation, from this date the University of Salamanca will contain an operational university library.

Trinity College Dublin houses the largest and oldest library in Ireland. Founded together with the University in the year one thousand five hundred and ninety-two, the Trinity Library contains over six million volumes printed with extensive collections of journals, manuscripts, maps, and music.

The Library holds the unique status of being able to request a free copy of every book published in the United Kingdom and Ireland. Among the books kept in Trinity's Library is the Book of Kells, proudly displayed by the University. The illuminated manuscript - dated around nineteenth century A.D. - was compiled by contributors from Colombian monasteries in Great Britain and Ireland. It contains the four Gospels of the New Testament.

Among the oldest libraries in the world, we must also consider the oldest library in the Americas, in Puebla, Mexico. It was founded in one thousand six hundred and forty-six by the then bishop of Puebla, Juan de Palafox y Mendoza, with the condition that anyone who was able to read had to be authorized to enter the Library.

In the year one thousand nine hundred and eighty-one, the Library was declared a Mexican National Historical Monument and in the year two thousand and five, UNESCO declared it a "Memory of the World" site. Today it remains open to everyone as a public library, in the spirit of Juan de Palafox y Mendoza.

Returning to Europe for a moment, the Queen's College Library in Oxford, United Kingdom, was founded together with the College in the year one thousand three hundred and forty-one by Robert Eglesfield, Chaplain to Edward the Third's wife, Queen Philippa.

Remaining in the United Kingdom, Trinity College houses the largest college library at the University of Cambridge. Like the College itself, Trinity's Library owes its foundation of one thousand five hundred and forty-six to King Henry the eighth.

The Library of Portuguese Literature in Rio De Janeiro was founded in the one thousand eight hundred and thirty-seven by Portuguese immigrants who wanted to promote European culture throughout Brazil. The construction of the library, however, did not begin before in the one thousand eight hundred and eighty.

Like the Library of Trinity College Dublin, this library has a rare arrangement whereby it receives a copy of every work published in Portuguese. Not surprisingly, the extraordinary collection of works is the largest collection of Portuguese literature outside of Portugal.

Originally founded by the Jesuits in the sixteenth century, the Clementium complex in Prague was officially recognized as a University in the seventeenth century, when the Library Hall was built. It remains the oldest library in the Czech Republic. According to legend, the Jesuits began their construction with only one book!

A small addition to this list for which we must thank one of our readers. The Chapter Library of Verona dates back to the fifth century AD, immediately after the Christianization of the city, which took place around three hundred and eighty.

It was precisely the religious men, in fact, that in the Middle Ages and even before the birth of the universities were involved in the preservation and production of texts. Among the oldest libraries in the world this is officially the oldest "in the area of Latin culture".

Endless rows of shelves, the scent of paper, silence: the world stops outside the large entrance doors, hundreds of other universes of ink and pages reign supreme inside.

Libraries are wonderful and fascinating places, almost sacred to some.

Which is the oldest book in the world?

It is difficult to say exactly what the oldest book in the world is. It is probably a part of the Bible, precisely the book of Genesis, which is thought to have been written more than three thousand five hundred years ago. The first modern book, printed with a modern printing press, is an edition of the Bible made in one thousand four hundred and fifty-five years ago by Johann Gutenberg, a German goldsmith and inventor from Mainz: it is thanks to his technique, called movable type printing, that books began to spread and cost less. In fact, they could be reproduced in many copies in a cheap and fast way. The pages of the Gutemberg Bible are decorated with drawings of plants and animals. Before this invention, the books were copied by hand, page by page, by the amanuensis, real specialists of writing.

Now that we have met the oldest, why don't we take another imaginary world tour to visit some of the most beautiful libraries in the world?

The first library I want to tell you about is the Royal Library of the Escorial Monastery, Madrid, Spain.

Wanted by Philip II, who wanted to gather here all the knowledge of the world, this library really leaves one speechless. Its painted ceilings are an exciting triumph of intense colors and frame thousands of masterpieces of literature.

The sacredness of this building is such that it almost seems to be in a cathedral. Simply beautiful.

A real European jewel is also the Royal Library in Copenhagen, Denmark. Known as a black diamond, this ultra-modern building in the port area of Copenhagen impresses with its elegance and simplicity. The interior and exterior of the library are in perfect and harmonious antithesis.

While the cold envelope of black marble and glass makes use of taut and sharp lines, in the interior, relaxing light, much more sinuous lines prevail.

In the heart of Europe, we also find the City Library in Stuttgart, Germany.

Inaugurated in October of the year two thousand and eleven, the city library of the automobile city is a true jewel of contemporary architecture.

Cold but not cold at all, this building stands nine floors high, and inside it is equipped with many comfortable spaces to enjoy the boundless number of books stored here. A joy for the eyes and the mind.

We stay in Germany to get to know another enchanted place: The Library of Wiblingen Abbey. Really beautiful the central hall: among the statues, the decorations, and the fantastic ceiling, you do not really know where to turn your eyes. The rooms of this library, which is now secularized, are a river of marble, colors, and gold.

On the other side of the ocean, we find the world-famous New York Public Library in New York, United States of America, also known for the Hollywood film industry, is one of the symbols of the city of New York and contains sixteen million books!

The beating heart of the building is the Rose Reading Room, which with its large crystal windows creates a muffled and incredibly special atmosphere.

Who does not remember the fairy tale of Beauty and the Beast?

I would like to conclude this imaginary journey through silently fascinating places by returning to the heart of Europe to get to know the wonderful library that was the protagonist of the scene in which Belle crosses the threshold of the spectacular library of the Beast's castle for the first time, until she falls in love with it. Well, that library, which made the protagonist of one of the most romantic fairy tales of all-time dream, really exists and is located in Austria.

The impressive library so beloved by the protagonist Belle is inspired by one of the most important historical convent libraries in Austria, near Linz, and seems to have come out of a fairy tale.

But what is the largest library in the world?

Located in Washington D.C., the Library of Congress is the national library of the United States and the largest in the world. Founded in the early nineteenth century, it contains materials in over four hundred and fifty languages, including one of the world's smallest books, Stradivarius violins, and some digitally archived tweets.

Isn't it wonderful and reassuring to be aware that you still have so many wonderful places to see in the world? There are not only amusement parks, breathtaking beaches, futuristic cities, there is and always will be a part of the world, like libraries, that will be preserved for future generations, so that the past is not lost and these sacred places continue to be a bastion of culture and civilization.

After so much having made you discover places so full of austere silence, it now seems normal to me to accompany you to a nice deep sleep, as is my custom, with a smile on your lips.

That is why I thought I would tell you now about some ghost-infested library stories. Ghosts? Yup, just some nice little spirits!

Incredibly famous is the Willard Library, in Evansville, Indiana, USA. The library is located inside a magnificent Victorian style building, a true Gothic masterpiece. It is said that inside the structure is around the one thousand nine hundred thirty-seven the ghost of a lady covered by a gray veil.

The ghost seems to be that of Mrs. Louise Carpenter, daughter of the founder of the library, Mr. Williard Carpenter.

Before his death, he stated that he would leave a large part of his estate to the library, which his daughter did not like so much that she sued him.

Louise, however, lost the case and this tormented her so much that her ghost, inclined not to give up her property, decided to live eternity in that very library which was once supposed to be hers.

The fluctuating and silent ghost has been nicknamed The Grey Lady and it seems that after all, it is not too irritating a presence, on the contrary, the frequenters and employees of the library, unanimously assert that it does not give any disturbance.

One notices its passage thanks to the strong scent of musk that it leaves behind, or because of the books, which it moves from time to time.

Sometimes, however, she is a bit spiteful, especially when she turns the lights on or off, or when she opens or closes the taps in the bathrooms.

The Parmly Billings Library is a public library serving Yellowstone County in Montana but also one of the most haunted libraries in America.

It is home to not just one spectrum, but many more.

Ghosts have been sighted such as a dark-haired woman in the basement, a man wearing jeans and work boots on the second floor, and a white figure moving outside the fifth-floor windows.

These apparitions are also accompanied by strange movements among the piles of books in the Montana room.

Uh, what a thrill...!

In the one thousand nine hundred and ninety-eight, Sharon Helfrich was hired as director at the Andrew Bayne Memorial Library, a public library in Bellevue, a suburb of Pittsburgh, Pennsylvania; since that day, this man claims to have witnessed numerous extraordinary events.

Lights and ceiling fans that go on and off, numbers that appear randomly on computer screens, shadows that move through the rooms, books that disappear and move on shelves, and a woman in Victorian dress who shows her disturbing presence.

What is the trigger for this episode? Apparently, Amanda Bayne Balph, former owner of the library, bequeathed it to the municipality in the year one thousand nineteen hundred and twelve, specifying that no tree on the property was to be cut down.

In the one thousand nine hundred and ninety-eight, however, when paranormal phenomena showed themselves in all their magnificence, an unfortunate fact happened. One of the trees in the residence, a three-hundred-year-old Dutch elm tree, died of an illness, which apparently gave way to the invasion of the ghosts.

Visitors to the Blanche Skiff Ross Memorial Library, Nevada, claim to have noticed paranormal phenomena such as books falling off shelves, carts rolling, and music audible on the back stairs.

In addition to this, the presence of an elderly man, wearing a jacket and cap, was noticed wandering around the balcony.

To keep him company, the ghosts of two girls in Victorian clothes playing carefree on the stairs, and a young woman in a long white dress reading a book, well, what else could she do in a library!

The Saline County Library in Benton, Arkansas, has not always been a library. From the sixties to the early twenty-first century, in fact, it was a theater in which, it was said, some ghosts lived.

Rotating carousels that moved by themselves, photocopiers that worked by themselves, doors that slammed without a particular reason, were evidence of the presence of ghosts.

One night, the director Julie Hart also happened to hear the sound of a typewriter running, which was strange since there were no typewriters left.

It is the belief of the place that the Peoria Public Library, located in Peoria, Illinois, was built on cursed ground. Just this would justify the presence of twelve ghosts!

The history of this library is not very cheerful, its first three directors died in unusual circumstances and the various employees claim to have been called while they were completely alone among the books.

They also claim to have been struck by cold air currents and that on the threshold of the basement you can see the face of one of the former directors.

In one thousand nineteen hundred and sixty-six the library was demolished, and another was built in its place. Although the building has changed, the employees continue to claim that ghosts are still in their place among the books.

According to patrons of the Pattee Library, Pennsylvania, inside the building, you can hear audible cries all the way to the basement of the building and see book carts moving quietly by themselves.

In addition to this, you can also catch a glimpse of transparent, red-eyed girls browsing through books. Who knows, maybe they must have been avid readers who spent the night reading instead of sleeping.

The Houston Public Library, Texas, is home to an incredibly special guest: the ghost of janitor Frank Cramer, who used to play his violin at night in the rooms of the library now closed to the public.

Cramer lived in the basement of the library and has never married there since his death in the Thirties. Inside the library, in fact, it is said that a spectral music is audible.

The Phoenixville Public Library, also in Pennsylvania, is home to three different ghosts.

One of them is an original lady who lives in the attic, dressed in a long antique dress and a very tall hat.

Among other things, she seems to be dropping books off the shelves.

Okay, we have come to the end, I would say we have had enough ghosts!

I close our scary excursus with the Scottsdale Public Library, Arizona, a place so special that it hosted a real investigation by an organization of professional ghost hunters.

The research team even found unjustifiable disappearances of books and things on the shelves but claims to be able to say that this is nothing of concern, just a search for attention by the people living there.

Among all the amazing libraries we have visited in this story, there should be some special place that you have been particularly impressed with, or maybe you would like to visit, or even just that you could imagine better. So, now imagine that you can enter this library.

It doesn't matter where it is, in what part of the world we are located, if it is cold if it is hot if it is raining outside or the sky is beautiful, these are details that don't make any difference.

Feel the soles of your shoes resonating on an old wooden beamed floor. From the high, decorated windows, the last rays of a golden, muffled, accommodating light come in through. Inside, the typical low and green lamps, those one similar to mushrooms, which turn on and off with the dangling chain only remain lit, those that are turned on and off with the chain dangling, which illuminate only a few volumes left open by some readers on huge solid wood tables.

You are enveloped by that magical and mystical smell of paper, the smell of fairytale books and stories that someone used to read to you when you were a child, that very good smell of quiet and satisfying moments.

You can wander a bit between the shelves, they are all sorted by genre, for example there is the area dedicated to science, history, mathematics, fiction, detective stories, biographies, thrillers, classics, the list is really endless, and in each genre you will find the authors arranged in alphabetical order.

Everything is ordered and in its place.

You can find everything you want, and you know that that book will always be there waiting for you.

But now is not the time to devote ourselves to long and stimulating readings, we are here to enjoy the most important feature of this place: silence.

Imagine that in libraries you can sleep.

Imagine that there is between the shelves, arranged to create a private and wonderfully comfortable area, a sort of personal refuge, an amazingly comfortable bed.

An unbelievably soft and inviting bed, already warm, scented of clean, ready for you.

You lift the flap of the sheets and put yourself in it, one leg at a time.

It is comfortable and cozy, and all around you are surrounded only by a perfect silence.

In the distance you can only hear some pleasant murmur of pages flipped through, people reading immersed in their thoughts, focused on stories and information capable of stopping the mind on distant things.

Turn the page too, turn on a blank sheet of paper.

This white sheet is your white pillow.

Let yourself go, don't think about anything anymore.

Inhale the magical scent of paper and relax.

There is an absolute silence, perfect for sleeping and having wonderful dreams.

Here time seems to have stopped.

Nobody runs, nobody talks fast, nobody can disturb.

You are perfectly comfortable here.

Feel the heavy eyes, feel the eyelids closing and sticking to the lower rhyme of the eye.

The breath becomes heavy and rhythmic.

It is okay, you have moved on and you can sleep in peace and serenity surrounded by culture and silence, reassured by a wonderful and relaxing place.

Let us be quiet, you sleep now.

The page is white.

Chapter 9 Slow as Snow

This story is a bit special, or at least I really wish it were.

To give you pleasant dreams and let you sleep peacefully, while I was telling you stories and legends, I used your power of visualization a lot. We imagined together wonderfully painted parks with the colors of autumn, Caribbean beaches, relaxing massages and melodic songs from enchanted mermaids, and even on this occasion I would like you to imagine yourself immersed in something beautiful and soothing to accompany you into the world of dreams with a smile on your lips.

It's Christmas time, it's a special Christmas, a Christmas without chaos or presents, it's just a perfect time when you don't have to rush to look for presents, you don't have to spend if you don't want to, you don't have to organize anything, imagine having a special moment reserved for you and you can enjoy a little bit of relaxation just for you.

You are at the window, a window decorated with typical Christmas lights, colorful ribbons, and some candles.

On the glass drops of condensation created by the internal warmth in reaction to low outside temperatures. You are sipping a hot drink, something you like very much and that warms your body.

You are admiring the snow, which slowly comes down from the sky whitening and absorbing colors and noises.

Winter gives us something else that the other seasons do not bring us: snow. It is undeniable as a beautiful snowfall, especially if unexpected, you give us the good mood. But how come?

Someone might object that snow doesn't bring us anything good: just a little is enough, and that immaculate mantle gets dirty, we need to clean the streets, free the cars, it takes longer to get to work, it slides easily on the ice and we could get stuck at home. It is true, there are negative aspects related to this meteorological phenomenon.

Yet even though the news of a snowstorm may initially worry us, a certain positive excitement takes over. The explanation lies in our emotional memory. When we remember some past events, the memory also brings with it the emotion associated with it. Our first experiences with the snow are undoubtedly joyful: getting up in the morning and discovering the snowy world meant not having to go to school, playing snowballs, making a snowman, etc... Those happy memories re-emerge easily in adulthood, and that is exactly how I would like you to feel right now.

Simply happy.

It is palpable the light-heartedness and joy that spread in the air thanks to a beautiful snowfall and adults allow themselves things that they would normally leave to children.

Just as schools close, snow often makes travel difficult, transportation is interrupted, and it is impossible to go to work. After the initial frustration, we can stop, watch the event from behind the windows, share our emotions with friends and family by sending photos and videos: the snow generates a break in routine, an unexpected vacation.

Now, you are enjoying that magical vacation.

Do you know that the snow is technically colored? Oh yes, and it is of all colors: frozen crystals reflect all the light, and we perceive it as white because white is the sum of all colors.

Snow is one of the greatest symbols of purity.

Looking at a snowy landscape has the power to calm us. This is also due to the characteristic of snow to absorb sounds. In fact, the snow cover is not compact: like whipped cream, between one flake and another there is air that, precisely because wrapped in ice, returns the muffled sounds. The effect is amplified because, usually, traffic tends to decrease and there are fewer people on the street.

That is why you feel wonderfully calm even now, while being comfortable in your armchair or warm under the blankets of your bed you are imagining a generous Christmas snowfall.

The snow offers a clean canvas where everything leaves a trace, like the passage of a bird or a cat.

You will be enchanted for a long time by the dance of the snowflakes on the ground.

You are in no hurry, no commitment, no one looking for you, calling you urgently, no worries.

Some snowflakes are really big, they seem soft, fluffy and very light, some others are very small, tender and cute.

Sometimes it is automatic: we approach the window; something attracts our attention, and we watch as time passes slowly and inexorably. Many people do it feeling a certain sense of guilt, they blame themselves for wasting time thinking that looking out the window is a passive act, which is useless. But that act of letting the eyes freely observe the landscape, while the wandering mind relaxes, is much more useful than we imagine.

Plato suggested that our ideas are like birds fluttering in the aviary of our brain. For birds to settle down, he considered that we need periods of calm without any particular purpose. Looking out the window gives us this opportunity, if there is snow outside this window then the effect is exhilarating!

Seeing the world go by while we are calm and relaxed is like getting off the train for a few minutes. We have no specific goal, and our attention wanders aimlessly, so the simple act of looking out the window can be almost as relaxing and restorative as meditation.

Standing in front of the window frees us from immediate pressures and worries, allowing the mind to wander freely.

So, let's get rid of all those absurd beliefs that impose certain actions as exclusively the property of the elderly, or slackers, because it is absolutely not the truth.

What if you feel like playing in the snow?
You can do it, just like when you were a child.

Being the first to draw on this canvas gives an undeniable satisfaction, like seeing our footprints as we walk. In addition, everything looks more vivid in front of the white coat and we notice the green of firs and other plants, the dark colors of the birds crawling around and all the creatures that, not living in the areas normally covered with snow, do not need to be light in color to camouflage themselves. Including humans.

Hey, how about making a nice snowman?

After all, what winter is without a snowman?

Big and small, kind and nice, with carrots instead of noses and an old bucket on the head, they are born, as if by magic, in the courtyards of towns and villages, lovingly shaped, rolled up by the hands of children and adults.

How many snowmen appear around us during the winter? Hundreds! Look at them and every time you are amazed by the imagination, shape, and originality of the "sculptors"!

Maybe you do not know it, but this cheerful winter idea has been known to people for more than a century. But not many people know what supernatural meaning the snowman had in the past...

According to an ancient legend, at the end of the fifteenth century, around one thousand four hundred and ninety-three, the sculptor, architect, Italian poet Michelangelo Buonarroti first sculpted a figure of snow.

According to historical research also, the first written mention of a snowman is found in a book of the eighteenth century: it talks about a giant "beautiful snowman". And the word "schneeman", which means "snowman", originally originated in the German language. The picture of a snowman first appeared as an illustration for a children's song book published in Leipzig.

The first snowmen were portrayed as cruel and ferocious snow monsters of impressive dimensions. It is no coincidence, because in those days' ancient ruthless winters with strong frosts and blizzards brought many problems. Most likely, it was then that the beliefs appeared, according to which snowmen pose a real threat to people. They thought it was dangerous to carve them during full moon periods: for a person, disobedience can turn into obsessive nightmares, night fears and indeed all kinds of failures. And in Norway there was a legend that it was dangerous to watch snowmen late at night. Also, meeting a snow figure at night was considered a bad sign: it was recommended to go around it.

Only in the nineteenth century the snow creatures became "kinder" and soon became an irreplaceable attribute of Christmas and New Year. Greeting cards with a smiling snowman surrounded by cheerful children quickly gained popularity.

It is curious that in the minds of European peoples, a snowman is always a male creature, they have never had snow women and snow maidens. In English, there is only one word for this: "snowman".

According to an ancient European parable, St. Francis of Assisi considered the creation of snowmen as a peculiar method to fight demons. And according to another Christian legend, snowmen are angels. After all, snow is a gift from heaven. This means that the snowman is nothing more than an angel who can transmit to God the requests of people. For this little snowman they shaped from the freshly fallen snow and silently whispered to him their wish. They believed that as soon as the snow figure melted, the wish would immediately be delivered to heaven and soon it would come true.

Snowmen have always been modeled near houses, richly decorated with garlands and household utensils, wrapped in scarves and branched brooms were delivered to their hands. In the details of their "clothing" one can guess a mystical character. For example, a carrot-shaped nose was attached to propitiate the spirits that send harvest and fertility. The bucket upside down on the head symbolized wealth in the house.

In Eastern Europe, the custom of decorating a snowman with "pearls" of garlic heads has long been known. It was believed that this promoted the health of families and protected them from the leprosy of dark power.

In Russia, snowmen have been shaped since ancient pagan times and revered as the spirits of winter. The Russian people to ask for help and to reduce the duration of heavy frosts have carved snowmen, unlike their European neighbors. The ancient inhabitants of Russia believed that female spirits ruled the natural winter phenomena such as fogs, snowfalls, blizzards, so to show them our respect, they carved snow women.

Today, in our civilized world, the creation of snow figures remains not only the favorite pastime of children, but also a socially organized vacation.

All over the world, they have also set records for sculpting the tallest snowmen. And the record for creating the world's tallest snowman was set in the United States of America in the year one thousand nine hundred and ninety-nine.

For each of us, what will be forever the most beautiful snowman in the world?

Obviously, ours! It will always be and will always remain the snowman that we made in that special moment, the one we remember with more pleasure, it could be the one made by children in the garden behind the house or the one made by adults with our kids.

However, it remains fixed the fact that every snowfall is a special occasion.

After playing with the snow, we return to observe what the snowy atmosphere and the magic of Christmas offer us, for example: the Christmas tree.

Who does not love Christmas trees?

The magic of decorating the tree in the family, or even alone with your own rhythms and ideas, and the thrill of seeing it all lit up and glittering is something that warms even the coldest and hardest hearts.

It is right around the Christmas tree that people gather on Christmas morning to unwrap the presents that have been placed at the foot of the tree. But where does the custom of decorating the fir tree for Christmas come from?

The origins of the Christmas tree are pagan. It seems in fact that at the origin of today's Christmas tree there is a long and ancient tradition that has its roots in Celtic culture. For the Druids, the ancient priests of the Celts, the fir tree was considered a symbol of long life, since it was always green even in winter. As winter approached, the firs were cut and decorated with ribbons, torches, small bells, and votive animals, to favor the spirits.

In addition to the Celts, it seems that the Vikings of the far north of Europe also followed the cult of the spruce tree, a tree capable of expressing magical powers. The trees were cut down, brought home, and decorated with fruits, recalling the fertility that spring would give them back.

With the birth of Christianity, the use of the Christmas tree also became established in Christian traditions. What gives it a Christian meaning is the biblical scene of Eden. On the night when the birth of Christ is celebrated, the tree in the center of the Garden of Eden also becomes the tree around which humanity finds forgiveness.

It seems that the Christmas tree was born in Tallinn, Estonia in the fifteenth century, when a large fir tree was erected in the Town Hall Square, around which young bachelors, men and women, danced together in search of their soul mate. The custom was then resumed in Germany, where towards the end of the sixteenth century a tree decorated in Bremen with apples, walnuts, dates, and card flowers is told. Among the cities that claim to be the home of the first Christmas tree, there is also Riga in Latvia, thus resuming the tradition in the Baltic countries, where there is also a plaque written in eight languages to commemorate the event.

With what colors is the house decorated for Christmas?
With the colors of tradition, reassuring and festive.

The inevitable is red: it is the pivotal color of the year-end celebrations, the inevitable from tree balls to flowers like the poinsettia. This color, typical of the aristocracy, for Christians is also chosen to recall the role of Jesus as the guide of all men. In addition, it is associated with the figure of Santa Claus or, more precisely, St. Nicholas, the saint most loved by children, also known as Samiklaus, Sinterclaus or Santa Claus. The saint was bishop of Myra and performed some miracles that allowed him to save children. Only at the end of the nineteenth century he began to be depicted dressed in red and with a white beard, and in the twentieth century American advertising agencies consecrated him to the iconography that we all know well and love so much.

Very present is also the green, which is the color of nature, abundance, the Earth that resists and offers its gifts despite the cold and winter frost. It is also the color of rebirth and resurrection.

Then there is the white of course, which is the gradation that indicates purity, as well as typical of the meadows and snowy fields at the end of the year.

And finally, there are the beautiful and luminous gold and silver, precious and noble colors, which represent light and their victory over darkness.

A must to decorate the branches of the tree are the traditional red balls. The choice of red apples as Christmas decoration is due on the one hand to the fact that their bright color stands out pleasantly on the green of the tree. Pine green and apple red are in fact imprinted in the collective memory as the colors of Christmas par excellence. The other reason that explains the choice of red apples was a reference to the tree of the Knowledge of Good and Evil in Eden. The apple recalled the forbidden fruit, symbol of Adam and Eve's original sin. The twenty-fourth of December in ancient times was celebrated the day of Adam and Eve. In the days preceding this now decayed feast, special theatrical performances were staged in the villages and towns. These performances were used to communicate to ordinary people, who often did not know how to read, the religious truths contained in the Bible.

Even today apples are still used as Christmas decorations. In Poland, Northern Europe, the Christmas tree is decorated with apples, oranges, candies, chocolates wrapped in colored paper, walnuts wrapped in foil. In northern Italy, Christmas trees are decorated with natural red apples, but also with flaked, sweetened, lacquered, caramelized apples. Not only that, but the house is also decorated with traditional and original decorations made with apples. In addition, many recipes of the Christmas period are based on apples.

In Wales is still widespread "Calennig", a decoration that is displayed in houses or donated to friends as a sign of good luck for the new year. It is made with an apple that is placed on a tripod made of twigs and stuck with abundant cloves. On the top, where the petiole stands, there is a boxwood twig decorated with raisins as if they were its fruits.

Over time, many other ways to decorate the tree have spread, Christmas tree decorations of all kinds, handmade Christmas balls, up to modern Christmas lights.

But it will be in France, and in particular in the Northern Vosges, in French Lorraine, that the first glass ornaments, produced by skilled glass masters, will be born.

I will tell you briefly how it went: it was the winter of one thousand eight hundred and fifty-eight in France, a winter that was particularly harsh and the red apple harvest had not been good. There were few apples, not even enough to support the people of those areas, and certainly there were not enough to decorate the Christmas Tree. It was then that a craftsman in the small village of Goetzenbruck, which had been home to a factory specializing in the production of watch glass since the beginning of the eighteenth century, had an original idea. Since in the manufacture of watch glass, the glass was cut into balls that were then blown, this gentleman thought that the glass balls could be blown to make sparkling decorations for the Christmas tree in the village. His idea was an immediate success, and immediately in Goezenbruck, in addition to optical glass, glass balls for the Christmas Tree were produced and soon exported all over the world.

What do we traditionally put at the foot of the tree? Christmas gifts.

Special gifts that should make us stop for a moment to think, gifts that should tempt us to make happy, if only for an ephemeral moment, the people we love the most.

The inhabitants of ancient Rome used to exchange gifts at parties and on New Year's Eve. This custom was linked to a tradition according to which, on the first day of the year, the king was offered as a gift a twig picked in the woods of the goddess of health. This auspicious rite spread among the people and soon, the twigs of laurel, olive and fig trees were replaced by various gifts.

Well, as you may have guessed by now, I am about to tell you more curious legends about what something is nowadays widespread and considered in all the world's populations and cultures.

Then we have a tender legend related to Christmas bells. At that time, shepherds flocked to Bethlehem as they traveled to meet the newborn king. A little blind child sat on the side of the main road and, hearing the announcement of the angels, begged passers-by to lead him to the Child Jesus. None had time for him, poor boy. When the crowd had passed and the streets were silent again, the child heard in the distance the slight ringing of a cattle bell. So, he thought: "Hey! Maybe that cow is in the stable where the baby Jesus was born!" and he followed the bell with determination to the stable where the cow took the blind baby to the manger where the newborn Jesus lay.

And the Advent Crown?

Well, it is an essential element of the preparation of Christmas in Germanic countries and

Scandinavian, where there is no home, church, or public place where there is no show.

It is a crown of welcome or good wishes and comes from an ancient pre-Christian tradition: in ancient times, it was customary to weave a wreath of evergreen leaves that represented the hope of a rebirth and this symbology has continued over the centuries until it spread among the Christian peoples and materialized in a crown of fir branches adorned with four candles, symbolizing the four weeks before Christmas, the period of Advent. The candles, traditionally purple in color, are lit every Sunday of Advent and each candle has a meaning: the candle of Bethlehem, the shepherds' candle, the prophets' candle and the angels' candle, until Christmas Eve, when the four lighted candles evoke the resurgence of light.

Could there not be a legend linked to the Holly?

A little orphan lived with some shepherds when the angels appeared announcing the happy news of the birth of Christ. On the way to Bethlehem, the child

woven a crown of laurel branches for the newborn king. When the little one placed it in front of Jesus, however, the crown seemed so unworthy to him that the shepherd boy was ashamed of his gift and began to cry. Then Baby Jesus touched the crown, made its leaves shine an intense green and changed the orphan's tears into red berries.

Could not miss the most authentic nature in traditional decorations, I am referring to the poinsettia, whose legend has its roots in Mexico.

In Mexico City, lived a poor little girl named Ines. On the evening of Christmas Eve, she wanted to bring a flower to the Baby Jesus but did not have the money to buy it. She went around the street without knowing what to do, then she decided to pick some twigs from a bush seen by chance among the ruins of a church. After picking them she decided to embellish the branches with the only beautiful thing she had: a red bow for her hair. She arrived at the church which was dark, and Ines thought she could find no one there. Once in front of the Baby Jesus, she laid down her bouquet. Immediately after putting it near the statue, she heard voices behind her: they were amazed and intrigued by the wonderful flower of Ines. Everyone started asking her where she had found such a beautiful flower. Ines turned to her bouquet and, incredulously, saw that the green leaves of the bush had turned red and the golden berries in the center had taken the shape of a heart. Ines returned home happy thinking that Jesus had liked her gift because she had transformed it into the most beautiful flower in Mexico: the poinsettia.

Another famous Christmas plant traditionally recognized as a good omen plant is mistletoe. Mistletoe embodies the spirit vital and is therefore protective since it has no ties with the earth and is also considered to be a panacea against all evils. Already Virgil in the Aeneid cites it for its magical virtues and also the Celts worshipped it as a sacred plant. The Druid priests when the winter solstice distributed to the people, who considered it a gift from heaven and believed in its effect. medicated. It is still customary today to donate a sprig of mistletoe as a symbol of good wishes for the new year.

Remaining on the theme of nature and interweaving with Christmas I also want to tell you the legend of the Robin.

At that time, a small brown bird shared the stable in Bethlehem with the Holy Family. At night, while the family was sleeping, it noticed that the fire was going out and soon the cold would come down, so it flew down to the embers and kept the fire alive with the movement of its wings all night long, to keep the baby Jesus warm. In the morning, the little bird discovered that he had been rewarded with a beautiful bright red chest as a symbol of his love for the newborn king.

Let's close this set of legends about what has always been the side dish of our Christmas with something sweet and delicious: dog candy, those inviting red and white candy canes, known among children who use them for Christmas tree decorations and not only... With a tasty and fresh mint flavor, the candy cane belongs to the Anglo-Saxon Christmas tradition that children receive and appreciate as sweets to lick and suck, as well as useful to decorate the tree along with cookies in the shape of bells and snowmen. Also, this lollipop has a beautiful legend of its own, full of meanings that is well suited to the Christmas period. It is said that an American confectioner wanted to invent a cake to be dedicated to Jesus, and just to remember him, he invented the stick, the shepherds' stick, J-shaped like Jesus, white in color, to signify the purity of Jesus, and red, to remember the blood he spilled. Today, sugar sticks are available in a myriad of different colors and flavors and are appreciated by Christians and non-Christians throughout the year.

I hope this set of Christmas curiosities made you smile.

But what I would like you to understand now is that Christmas is not only December, but it also doesn't have to be linked to winter, traditions or its religious significance. Christmas can and must be a time of celebration and rebirth for all of us.

It can be Christmas every day if we want it to be, we can return happy children at any time. Of course, we are adults, we can't pretend we don't have stressful days that wear us out physically and psychologically, but it takes just a moment to try to push away anxiety and depression and finally find within us the relief we so desire.

You know, sometimes it is enough to sit near a window and stop thinking allowing the gaze to wander and the mind to break a moment to catch up. We can do this anywhere, at home, in the office, on the train, at the doctor's, at school, sitting at a diner. No matter what's out there, it's normal that unfortunately we won't always be able to find ourselves in front of postcard landscapes, we might find ourselves on a busy road instead of a snow-whitened garden with a beautiful snowman waving at us in the middle or along a paradisiacal beach; the important thing is the action as an end in itself.

Right now, it is not necessary for you to get up from your comfortable position to go and look out a window, you can very well use that superpower I taught you to use: visualization.

Let's take the image with which we opened this story:

Imagine sitting comfortably and warmly next to a beautiful window.

You have just finished sipping a hot drink, your favorite, tea, chocolate, milk, whatever you prefer.

Outside the snow falls slowly, the flakes of ice crystals dance festively from the sky until they settle like feathers on the earth.

All sounds are muffled, and every form of animal and earthly life is enveloped in the pure whiteness of white.

The house is full of Christmas decorations, and you now know a bit of stories about the elements that traditionally accompany the festivities and you can impress others if you want.

A beautiful fire burns and crackles in the fireplace, spreading a pleasant and enveloping warmth and a magical sound of wood and embers.

You have a soft blanket on your shoulders, you are warm and safe.

You feel great, nothing is wrong. Inside you, it is Christmas.

Put your forehead to the wall next to the window and close your eyes, you really want to get a good night's sleep.

All the lights are off, the house is lit only by the fire in the fireplace and the warm and colorful Christmas tree lights.

If you like them, you can imagine in the background typical Christmas carols or a light sound of bells, such as those related to Santa's reindeer sleigh.

Sleep now, have sweet dreams, golden and silver dreams, red, white, and green, tomorrow morning will be the day of rebirth and relief.

Sleeping will make you feel better, but remember to always carry Christmas inside you, and never forget to feel like a happy child again.

Good night.

Conclusion

And so, page after page, we came to the end of this book.

We have been on a long journey together, and I sincerely hope I have been able to make you feel better. My real intention was to accompany you as a guide in the world of dreams and teach you some methods and cues to relax and let you go to a moment of total relaxation and inner peace.

I would like to know that maybe at the end of a stressful day or in the middle of a complicated meeting at work, you would find relief in rethinking some of the stories we lived together in the previous pages.

Remember that if you don't have the right mindset inside you and total confidence in what is contained in this book, something may not work, and sleep will find many obstacles on its way to you. Health comes first, and healthy sleep is essential at all ages and for all people, regardless of who they are, what they do, where they go and where they come from. Trust me, sleep is the foundation of individual well-being.

If this book, as I hope it will, has helped you achieve the goals for which you chose it, I would be very grateful if you would leave me your opinion in a review so that I can know if I did a good job or not and maybe induce some other stressed adult with anxiety problems, insomnia and difficulty falling asleep, to find a way to fall asleep with a smile on his lips.

Thank you from the bottom of my heart.

This has been:

Bedtime Stories for stressed Out Adults

Learn the Power of Visualization, Relieve Worries, Reduce Anxiety, Heal Insomnia, and Fall Asleep Deeply with a Smile.

Written by **Diana Shelby**

CPSIA information can be obtained
at www.ICGtesting.com
Printed in the USA
LVHW021305040121
675400LV00004B/431